BROTHER DOCTOR

By

Albert Arkhim Gewargis, M.D.

Co-written by
Lynn Santer

First published in 2006
by Poseidon Books
http://www.poseidonbooks.com
An imprint of Zeus Publications
P.O. Box 2554,
Burleigh M.D.C. QLD. 4220
Australia

The National Library of Australia Cataloguing-in-Publication

Gewargis, Albert Arkhim, M.D.
Brother doctor.

ISBN 1 921118 94 6.

1. Gewargis, Albert Arkhim, M.D. 2. Physicians – Iraq – Biography. 3. Kurds –
Iraq. I. Santer, Lynn, 1961- . II. Title.

610.92

BROTHER DOCTOR

By Albert Arkhim Gewargis, M.D.

Co-written by Lynn Santer

Non-fiction bio epic of the Herculean and heroic
mission of mercy in Kurdistan
by
By Doctor Albert Arkhim Gewargis

Poignant and heart-rending, inspirational and tragic.

In 1970 a treaty was signed.

In 1974 the treaty was broken,
and the genocide began.

Today it's time the world learned the truth.

Dedicated to my father, Arkhim, and wife, Isolde

I am humbled and grateful beyond words for all my father gave up for me. Despite regular beatings at the hands of Saddam Hussein's brutal thugs my father's spirit, his belief in and love for me, and his determination to live to see a free Iraq never died. I owe him a debt I can never repay. I owe him my very life. It is a great tragedy that he passed away while I was still in the mountains of Kurdistan. In human flesh I could never say thank you or good-bye. Instead I say this to him now, "Father, in this book your memory, and your sacrifice, will be immortalized so that future generations may know how great a man Arkhim Gewargis was."

My wife, Isolde, has been my living breathing inspiration and strength. When the night was blackest, and the visions of despair their brightest, Isolde stood by my side and held my hand encouraging me to tell my story. I love you with all my heart, mind, body and soul, Isolde, and I always will.

SYNOPSIS

This is a real life story of courage and despair in proportions that eclipse anything you have ever before read – or even imagined. It's a tale of tragedy and triumph against the most brutal circumstances any human being could begin to conceive. And it's a journey of heroism and horror that rivals the most spectacular myths of legend, because every word of it is true.

Doctor Albert Arkhim Gewargis was raised in Iraq as an Assyrian Christian. He completed his medical degree in Germany, where he lived on a year-by-year visa until the heinous bombing of the Israeli Olympic team in Munich, 1972. Forced to leave Germany for no other reason than he was a citizen of Iraq, Albert decided to return to his homeland, despite persecution, and despite the fact that he had the opportunity to live in several other countries of the world.

With war looming between the Kurds and the Ba'ath Party of fascist Iraq, this brave and dedicated man of medicine gave up everything to help a people who had touched his heart.

Don't read this book because you sympathize with the plight of the Kurdish people. Don't even read this book because you condemn the sadistic tyranny of Saddam Hussein's Ba'athist regime. Read this book to be inspired by the endurance and determination of one man who was so dedicated to saving lives that he voluntarily faced squalor and starvation, physical and mental agony, and torment and frustration that would have sent a lesser man insane.

The first building Albert was assigned to use as a hospital had previously been used as a stable. Two tons of dung had to be dug out, and DDT saturated throughout the complex to rid it of rats, poisonous snakes, scorpions, and malaria carrying mosquitoes, before he could begin to operate.

Often he had no food to eat, and no bed to sleep in. He could have left at any time. Indeed Doctor Gewargis had no obligation to be there in the first place. Yet he remained, moved by the haunting sound of a child singing in angelic tones under sedation as his arm was being amputated, dazed by the ninety-year-old guerrilla who shouted encouragement to his men as Albert treated his gaping wounds without anesthetic, and crushed when he arrived in a remote area of Iraqi Kurdistan to deal with a measles outbreak only to find seventy freshly dug little graves.

He was bombed, he was shot at, and he walked for days to help others until his feet were in bleeding shreds. His story begins over a decade in advance of the grim fate that awaited the Kurdish people of Iraq … the holocaust known as 'Bloody Friday' where Saddam Hussein used his devastating weapons of mass destruction on a simple people who wanted nothing more than to defend their right to exist.

BROTHER DOCTOR

PREFACE

This is the story of a people who truly live up to the meaning of their name, the Pesh Merga, 'We who face death'.

In an area of Iraq little known by most of the Western world, a brave and proud people faced annihilation at the hands of one of the most ruthless dictators the world has ever known. While you may think you know the story, the truth is more steeped in antediluvian history and more shocking than the worst annals of war crimes in the chronicles of humanity. While people in homes around the globe drank their morning coffee the systematic genocide of an ancient race was not only being planned with vile and malevolent audacity, it was actually being carried out. This atrocity, for the main part, managed to slip totally under the radar of international media. This is not the story of the gassings that you know about. This is the lead up to those events that took place years before most of the Western world even knew a place called Kurdistan existed.

This tale will take you on an odyssey as witnessed through the eyes of the people themselves. You will learn, perhaps for the first time, what these noble villagers were truly fighting for. And you will journey through some of the most breathtakingly beautiful mountains and valleys on earth, those which provided the backdrop for this most unholy of wars. My personal experience intertwines with thousands of these people, including the Kurdish guerrillas known as 'the Pesh Merga'. It is these people whose name means, 'We who face death'.

This story is about a brutal crusade against a people who were doing nothing more than defending their right to exist. It is the story of suffering and oppression in a barbaric conflict, the outcome of which seemed pre-destined and devastating even before the battle had

1

begun. But perhaps most importantly, it is a story that cannot reach a happy conclusion before the outside world understands who these people really are.

In the province of Sulaymaniyah, a small but very important part of Kurdistan, there is a highway between two Kurdish cities. Iraq is full of such highways, highways where Iraqi military garrisons attacked without mercy, killing, maiming, and sending frightened children running into the freezing and unforgiving night. Before my odyssey into Iraq ended, the towns and small villages that once lay peacefully in this idyllic landscape were deserted or destroyed. In amongst this insanity there was a frontline hospital staffed by those who would not turn and run. And there was an outsider working alongside these gallant people – me.

I began documenting this story over thirty years ago. It remained unfinished, unable to be told, for I was waiting for the struggle to be won, waiting until the cemeteries no longer resonated with the melancholy music of those in anguish for their beloved brethren who would never sing again. But now I know the tragic and complete story must be told. The information contained in the following pages is the tale of real people – the people who lived and died as actual players in this ghastly reality show. The events, the mountains, the valleys, the Pesh Merga, the hospital, and what we overcame and achieved is true even to the smallest detail.

Thirty years ago I was waiting for the happy ending to put to this story. In truth I was also afraid to publish my journal because so many members of my family lived in Iraq. Even today, when Saddam Hussein is no longer in power, there is still great fear of his criminal gangs. But the merest of lights now shines in Iraq; a light that brings the potential of a free future for all peoples in its land. In 1975, when the Ba'ath Party was at the peak of its power, this publication could not have been considered. It is not without risk today, but I can no longer remain silent. It is time to tell the truth.

I should point out that I am not a Kurd myself. I am Assyrian. Often when I tell people I am Assyrian, they reply, "A Syrian?" No, I am not a Syrian, I am an Assyrian, and I probably need to put that in its historical perspective...

Around 1380 BC, the Assyrians virtually came to control Babylonia, where they ruled for around two centuries. The Assyrian culture showed skill in science and mathematics from the beginning. Among the great mathematical inventions of the Assyrian people was definition of the circle into 360 degrees. They were also among the first to invent longitude and latitude.

In the 6th century BC, Nebuchadnezzar destroyed Jerusalem and took an estimated 15,000 captives, sending most of the rest of the population into exile in Babylonia. Ironically, perhaps, it was this blood-thirsty monarch who is credited with creating the fabled Hanging Gardens of Babylon, one of the seven wonders of the ancient world. Nonetheless, in the year 612 BC the capital city of Assyria, Nineveh, fell in burning plunder. Various invaders conquered the land after Nebuchadnezzar's death, including Alexander the Great in 331 BC. It wasn't until the 7th century AD that Arab Muslims captured it, and offered the inhabitants an ultimatum: "Accept the faith or love death as you love life." Most of the tribes were Christian at the time of this Islamic conquest.

Assyrians as an ethnic group suffered their share of hardships throughout history, and certainly in more recent times at the hands of Saddam Hussein. Hussein and his former Ba'ath regime carried out 'ethnic cleansing' by coerced relocation of indigenous Assyrians from their ancestral homelands, the outright suppression of the Assyrian ethnic identity, and the imprisonment, torture, and even execution of numerous Assyrian rights activists. The Assyrians lived side-by-side with the Kurds and the Turcoman. I am proud to be Assyrian, but I consider the Kurds 'my people' too – I feel a kinship for them, indeed I love them.

Kurdistan is comprised ethnically and religiously of Kurds (who are mainly Sunni Muslims), Assyrians (who are Christians), and Turcomans (who are also mainly Sunni Muslims). I shall explain more about the Kurdish history in Chapter Two. For now it is only important that you understand while I was raised in Iraq, and I consider myself kin to the Kurds, I am an Assyrian Christian.

Despite the horrific human rights abuses conducted against Iraq's Kurdish minority by the Ba'ath regime, the fact remains that Kurds were officially recognized as an Iraqi ethnic group alongside the Arab majority. Sadly the same cannot be said of Iraq's other ethnic groups, including both the Assyrians and the Turcomans, whose ethnic identity was blatantly denied under Hussein's reign. In fact in the censuses of 1977 and 1987, Assyrians and Turcomans were forced to register as either Kurd or Arab.

So, now you have a brief historical perspective of Assyrians, I should perhaps explain how I came to care for the Kurdish people during the Ba'athist holocaust...

CHAPTER ONE

It began in Munich:

I'd left my home in Iraq to study medicine in the USA and subsequently Germany, where I received my license to practice medicine. I was working at a hospital in Bavaria when the summer Olympics came to Munich in 1972. The Bavarian Alpine region town hospital was picked out as a shadowy outline against the drab sky. The early morning mists of a year that was moving towards autumn rose over a nearby lake, curtaining off the line of mountains behind them. Despite the early hour there was movement around the building. While the town was still largely dozing in continued sleep, the cars of busy hospital professionals drove away and others came to the car park to take their place.

I entered the building with many others to undertake my daily tasks as I had done every day for months before, the tasks of assistant doctor in a German hospital fitting in precisely with my ethos. I'd had no problem obtaining my medical license to practice following a successful study of medicine in the USA and Germany. Young qualified doctors were in great demand in Bavaria. Doors opened wherever I went with my applications, until an entirely unexpected event cancelled out everything I'd developed to date.

As I prepared for my round of the wards that morning, a shocking news report on the radio did not appear to be of immediate relevance to my fate. I heard a threateningly dark and distant announcer's voice coming from the radio in the neighboring nurses' room:

"Good morning. Tuesday the 5th of September, 1972. This is a special news bulletin replacing our standard news programs. A major hostage drama has occurred at the Munich Olympic Village in the early hours of the morning. The Israeli Olympic Team has apparently

5

been attacked in their accommodation by a Palestinian terror group.
It has not been possible to establish how many hostages are in the
hands of terrorists. Details of the event are not yet known."

The seriousness of the situation became ever clearer as the day wore on. Programs on the terror attack at the Olympic Village in Munich were broadcast on every radio station. From the first comments of German and Israeli politicians, it was possible to recognize a virtually complete and shame-faced helplessness of those responsible for law and order; they had apparently been taken completely by surprise. The names of the terrorists were mentioned unexpectedly, negotiations took place, and one deadline followed another. Persons offered themselves as alternative hostages. The focus of attention changed from the Olympic Village to the Airport Fürstenfeldbruck. The terrorist demands were apparently accepted. A Boeing 727 jet airliner was ready to depart on the runway, from where the terrorists wanted to fly with the hostages to Cairo. Helicopters brought them from the Olympic Village to the airport, but as they sought to board the aircraft it became obvious that the German government had no intention of allowing the terrorists to leave with their hostages.

Snipers were in position with the order to shoot to kill. A two-hour gun battle was fought between these snipers and the Palestinians before one terrorist's hand grenade exploded. The results of this deeply shocked those who were responsible as all eleven hostages, five terrorists, and one policeman were killed. The event changed forever the political landscape of Europe and the world.

The following day I was busy assisting in an operation as a secretary entered the operating theater in contravention of the clear rules. My concentration was so deeply on my work that I only noticed this as the chief surgeon demanded angrily, "What is this? Why are you disturbing us?"

"Please excuse me," the embarrassed young lady replied. "The people from the criminal investigation department are outside. They want to interview the assistant doctor."

"What? This can't be serious. We are in the middle of an operation."

"I have already told them, but they insist."

"This is the absolute end," the chief surgeon boomed, with a razor-sharp and searching glance in my direction.

"I don't have the least idea what's going on," I mumbled, a little dazed.

"Ah, you don't understand. But the police do. They must have an absolutely urgent reason for an action like this."

"But I don't understand," I insisted. "What should I do?"

"Listen to what they have to say. The criminal investigation department wants to speak to you, and what they have to say is clearly so important that they have no qualms about interrupting an operation."

"What does that mean? Should I go?" I asked feebly.

"Go!" the chief surgeon snapped angrily.

What I heard from the two plain-clothed policemen completely dumbfounded and confounded me: "You are to be ordered out of the country. You have precisely one week to arrange your departure for yourself otherwise you will be deported."

I could not believe what I was hearing.

"Why?" I blurted. "What have I done?"

"It is not our job to give you further information about these matters. All that we can tell you is contained in this document."

With those words one of the officers passed me a letter from the Bavarian Ministry of the Interior describing me as a risk to the inner security of the Federal Republic of Germany, confirming that I would have to leave Germany within a week. The officers left me with these parting words: "If you do not comply with this request then we shall be obliged to take deporting you into our own hands."

'Request' seemed a strange word to use for what was apparently a demand, although I still had difficulty processing the fact that this demand was in any way final.

"This is an error. There must be some mistake," I insisted.

But it was no mistake. A few hours later I had been sacked from my job without a word of thanks for the work I had put in. Neither my superiors nor my colleagues showed the least interest or sympathy for my situation, probably seeing me as a sympathizer with the terrorists, merely because I was originally from Iraq. I sought help with the local political representative, but there too it was as though I stood before a blank wall. All I could achieve was a minor extension to the ejection process; a deadline now of a generous two weeks. Deeply angered, I realized that in the tense political climate prevailing since the Munich hostage situation just being an Iraqi citizen was enough of a crime to warrant punishment and deportation.

I had left my parents' home in Iraq in the early 1960s to study abroad. Although I could have made a home in many countries when I was expelled from Germany, including the USA and other European countries, I decided it was time to return to my home in the Middle East. I would by no means be safe and free once I arrived there, on the contrary. Not only was I not a member of the ruling Ba'ath Party, and nor would I become one, but even worse I had made my opposition to Saddam Hussein and the brutal regime that ruled in Iraq very well known as part of the Iraqi student movement in Europe. These facts would put me firmly on the radar of Saddam Hussein's henchmen. Despite all this I wanted to return to Iraq. It was not an easy choice, but my decision was firm. I wound up my affairs, asked for my papers from the authorities, terminated my rental contract and left Germany a few days later from Frankfurt, before the deadline had even expired.

My brother awaited me – a deeply concerned man.

The fact that I was an experienced doctor counted for nothing in Iraq. I had to retake the State examinations, in themselves not easily granted to those who were not members of the Ba'ath Party. I kept a low profile for an entire year, hidden away at my parents' house in Baghdad. The route to a job in a hospital only opened to me after successfully completing my examinations a second time, and since I was not a member of the Ba'ath Party I had to appear before a government medical commission to decide which hospital I would be allowed to work in. I was presented with a list of country hospitals that were considered suitable for non Ba'ath Party members. None of the important hospitals in Baghdad or the south were on the list, but fortunately for me Sulaymaniyah hospital was. The members of the commission could not have expected what a blessing this was to prove for me, as I had already privately made the decision to disappear among the mountains in the north, to join an opposition group.

Baghdad was once a wonderful city, dignified by a millennia-old civilization, the capital of the Biblical land of two rivers, filled with oriental treasures. It was the 'Cradle of Mankind', well it was once. What had happened to this great city? It had become a place of terror and oppression, a city full of sad people, a single giant and brutal prison. Working in Baghdad did not appeal to me in the least!

I should explain when I was expelled from Germany I did not have German citizenship; rather I had been living in Germany under a work visa that I had to renew annually. When the Israeli Olympic team fell victim to that heinous act of terrorism, the German government reacted both swiftly and emotionally to the fact that Jews had been killed on their soil. Many who didn't hold German citizenship, and were from a remotely 'suspect' background, were immediately expelled from the country – it was nothing personal to me. Somewhere between five and six thousand people were thrown out of Germany that year, so in opting to return to Iraq my best hope was that my name might get lost somewhere in the crowd. I considered going to Beirut for a time, but I had family in Iraq whom I missed very much, and as a headstrong youth I decided the desire to see my family was more powerful than the risk of being killed by Saddam if I returned.

Deep in my heart the north of Iraq was truly the only place I wanted to be. It was the best place I could put my skills and talents to good use, back with the people I called my kin – the Kurds. I plunged myself headlong into the thousands of years-old struggle of the Kurdish people as they continued their fight for freedom. In ancient Kurdish legend the tale is told of an evil tyrant who prayed at the shrine of two serpents, that he fed with the brains of his Kurdish subjects, until one of those subjects rose up and called all the people of his village to join him. Together they stormed the palace of the evil tyrant and crushed the tyrant's head under a massive hammer, bringing the reign of terror to an end. From that point on the Kurds celebrated the first day of spring as 'Newroz', meaning 'new day'. The eternal attempt to conjure the 'Newroz' began for me in June, 1973. I literally 'headed for the hills', the mountains of Kurdistan, to a place where my destiny awaited…

9

CHAPTER TWO

To the casual observer the mountains of Iraqi Kurdistan could have leapt straight from the pages of a fantasy fairytale, seemingly candy-covered towers streaked by remnants of pure white snow reflecting golden sunbeams over miles of sweet-smelling purple flowers. The idyllic landscape of these ancient monuments provided an imposing backdrop for a small boy peering out from behind a rock. I watched as the boy screwed up his nose trying to shut out billowing wisps of smoke transfusing a sickening aroma of death unerringly into his nostrils, the scent of his burning village inescapable even in his dreams.

Every man, every woman, and every child in Kurdistan knew the history of their people, a history that has seen them endure forced relocations and war as far back as anyone could remember. Stoic and tough, many would use a year's savings to rent mules in order to escape the tyranny that seemed to follow wherever they would set up home. Many more would carry children too tired to walk any further, children who often became separated from their mothers in the panic and confusion of another exodus for these brave people. Yet despite exhaustion their morale and will to survive remained high. Those with food would feed those who had none. Lost children were cared for by complete strangers. While the West worried about their petrol prices going up, bewildered refugees could do little but wait for others to decide their fate. Weak as a result of being politically divided between Russia, Turkey, Iran, Iraq and Syria, the Kurds were oppressively ruled everywhere except for twenty-five thousand square miles in the mountains of Northern Iraq. The nations that ruled over the Kurds, traditionally at odds with one another, all united on one issue – their opposition to Kurdish independence.

The easiest way to attack these mountain people, who had no anti-aircraft guns, was to bomb them. This drove the people into mountain caves where hunger and disease finished the job. Polio, malaria, tuberculosis, meningitis, and typhoid were powerful allies for the Iraqi forces at a time when infant mortality for the Kurds was running at around thirty-five percent. It was a David and Goliath struggle, but against these odds one man emerged as a hero for the Kurdish movement to follow, Masoud Barzani. Masoud Barzani was born in Mahabad on the same day that the KDP (the Kurdish Democratic Party) was founded. At that time his father, General Mustafa Barzani, was Chief of the military of the Kurdish Republic of Mahabad. It was August 16th, 1946, when Quazi Mohammad, after rising to power in free elections, declared a Kurdish Republic in Mahabad within Iranian Kurdistan. In Masoud's own words "I was born in the shadow of the Kurdish flag in Mahabad and I am ready to serve and die for the same flag".

When the Republic fell, Mustafa Barzani went to the USSR with five hundred of his devoted followers. Masoud Barzani, the rest of the family, and thousands of Barzani clan members returned to Iraq and were promptly deported to the southern parts of the country. Masoud Barzani was twelve-years old when he was finally reunited with his father. Over time, the family moved back to their home village of Barzan, only to find it in ruins. Shortly thereafter, the Iraqi government resumed its repression against the Kurdish people. Left with no other alternatives, Mustafa Barzani and the KDP launched their armed struggle in 1961 to defend the rights of the Kurds.

At the age of sixteen, Masoud Barzani sacrificed his education and joined the Pesh Merga forces. The young Barzani was deeply influenced by the valor, leadership skills and compassion of his father. Masoud Barzani's experiences in the rugged mountains of Kurdistan were to provide him with the mettle and leadership skills that were to later propel him to the helm of the Kurdish movement.

It was not long before the KDP leadership began to notice the younger Barzani's qualities. It therefore came as no surprise when he, together with his elder brother, Idris, took part in the delegation

11

which signed the now defunct autonomy deal with Baghdad in March 1970. When the Iraqi government reneged on its pledges once again, the Kurdish armed struggle resumed. Once again Masoud Barzani took part at the side of his father until the end of the movement in 1975.

When KDP re-organized itself in 1976, Barzani was in the USA for medical treatment. Towards the end of 1978, he survived an assassination attempt in Vienna while returning to Kurdistan, where he assumed a leading position in the KDP with his brother Idris and other key figures. After the death of Mustafa Barzani in March 1979, Masoud was elected as the new president of the KDP in the 9th Party Congress. Since then he has been re-elected as the Party's President in three other general congresses.

For the Kurdish people war has always been the continuation of diplomacy by other means. Poor communications, economic blockades, and a land-locked frontier meant the wounded had a particularly tough time. Perhaps for this reason a foreign reporter once commented that the most important thing he saw during his tour of the 1974 conflict was my modest little frontline hospital. I am not ashamed to admit that the Kurdish people touched my heart and my soul. Their hospitality and generosity is a matter of honor that dates back far into Kurdish folklore. An old Kurdish proverb says, "It is better to lose property than to lose honor". Yet despite being tough, these people maintained a gentle streak that has prevented the cancer of fanaticism and political extremism developing. Sadly this chivalrous attitude was unhelpful in a world that had become accustomed to terrorism from otherwise impotent minorities as a fact of life.

The experience of the Kurdish people through the centuries has brought them little but poverty and subjugation, massacres and humiliation. These tragedies they have endured with unflinching courage and determination. The Kurds are the living embodiment of the idea that it is impossible to crush a nation which insists on freedom and is prepared to pay for its freedom at any cost. The Kurds, an Iranian ethno-linguistic group like Persians, Lurs, Baluch and Bakhtiari, inhabit the mostly mountainous area where the borders of Turkey, Iran, Iraq, and Syria meet. Following World War I and the breakup of the Ottoman Empire, the Kurds were promised their own country under the terms of the 1920 Treaty of Sevres only to find the offer rescinded under the 1923 Treaty of Lausanne. Numbering at least 25 million people, Kurds are mostly divided among Turkey, Iraq, Iran and Syria. The main area they inhabit is about 230,000 square miles, equal to German and Britain combined. The Kurds are the largest ethnic group in the world without a state. The term "Kurdistan" is widely used in Iraq to refer to the Kurdish area of northern Iraq and in Iran to refer to the Kurdish area of northwest Iran. Turkey and Syria, however, avoid this term for political reasons, although under the Ottomans it was widely used.

The area of northern Iraq where Kurds prevail is a region of about 83,000 square kilometers. This is about the same size as Austria. Smaller ethno-linguistic communities of Assyrian-Chaldeans, Turkomans, Arabs, and Armenians are also found in Iraqi Kurdistan. In Iraq there are approximately 3.7 million Kurds in the predominantly Kurdish northern safe haven area, and between one and two million in the rest of Iraq, particularly Baghdad, Mosul and that part of Iraqi Kurdistan still under the control of the Baghdad regime.

The majority of Kurds are Sunni Muslims. There are also Shi'a and Yezidi Kurds, as well as Christians who identify themselves as Kurds. Yezidis are Kurds who follow a religion that combines indigenous pre-Islamic and Islamic traditions. The once thriving Jewish Kurdish community in Iraq now consists of a few families in the Kurdish safe haven.

Since the creation of the modern state of Iraq, the history of Iraqi Kurdistan has been one of underdevelopment, political and cultural repression, destruction, ethnic cleansing and genocide. Al-Anfal (The Spoils) was the codename given to an aggressive, planned, military operation against Iraqi Kurds. It was part of an ongoing, larger campaign against Kurds because of their struggle to gain autonomy within the Republic of Iraq. Anfal took place during 1988 under the direction of Ali Hasan al-Majid, Saddam Hussein's cousin. He became known as "Chemical Ali" because of his use of chemical and biological weapons on Kurdish towns and villages.

The broad purpose of the campaign was to eliminate resistance by the Kurds by any means necessary. Its specific aim was to cleanse the region of "saboteurs"--who included all males between the ages of 15 and 70. Mass executions were carried out in the targeted villages and surrounding areas. The operation was carefully planned and included identifying villages in rebel held areas, declaring these villages and surrounding areas "prohibited" and authorizing the killing of any person or animal found in these areas.

Economic blockades were put onto these villages to cut them off from all support. The army also planned for the evacuation of them and the inhabitants' relocation to reservation-like collective towns. People who refused to leave were often shot. In some cases, people who agreed to leave were gathered up and separated, with men from 15 to 70 in one group; women, children, and elderly men in another. Many of the men were executed while the others were removed to the collective towns or to camps in the south of Iraq.

It was May 1973 when I received my assignment to work in the government hospital in Sulaymaniyah, one of the more important cities in Iraqi Kurdistan. I went first to Kirkuk, where I hired a car to drive the remaining one hundred and ten kilometers. The road was paved and smooth, running through an infinite landscape rich in the picturesque hues of nature. For the first time since leaving Baghdad I witnessed undulating pastures, all neatly ploughed and planted. Somehow I felt different. I felt free for the first time since I had returned to the place of my birth. Baghdad was once a beautiful city, but now it was nothing more than a city of horror and oppression, a city of sad people, a city which had effectively been turned into one giant prison.

On my way to Sulaymaniyah I suddenly realized I was finally going to have the chance to do something I had always dreamed of. I had a chance to do something meaningful, something real. I gazed with wonder and anticipation towards the impressive mountains ahead, feeling all the sensations of weakness and fear I'd experienced in Baghdad vanish like a morning mist. It was a sense of freedom such as I'd never known before. These cheerful thoughts were still drifting through my mind when three armed men stepped out from

14

behind some large rocks and waved at my car to stop. That was my introduction to the Pesh Merga. They were young men, all wearing the famous Kurdish khaki dress. Each one had a rifle, a full belt of ammunition, and their heads were covered with the Kurdish turban of the Sulaymaniyah region. I offered them cigarettes but they refused saying, "Zor spass kaka". Apparently these men were going to be traveling with us.

When we arrived at Jamjamal, we stopped in front of a teahouse on the main street and the three Pesh Mergas went their own way. Both the café and the streets were crowded with armed Pesh Merga, but in no way did I feel threatened by this. On the contrary, I felt a deep joy and true peace being among so many partisans. Actually at that time the Pesh Mergas were not true guerrillas, they were more like border guards, paid by the central government to keep law and order.

After a brief stop, I continued on to Sulaymaniyah, the scenery becoming wilder and greener with each mile I progressed. Soaking in the charm of villages that had remained virtually unchanged over centuries, I remember feeling a sense of home-coming. It never occurred to me that war could come within a thousand miles of this enchanting place. As I passed bazaars of delightfully vibrant stalls, I noticed the streets were busy with loud honking cars and the sidewalks crowded with bustling people, most of whom wore the vividly colorful Kurdish national costume. The bright bursts of joyful clothing in a stage set by destiny to bestow so much misery and hardship left me with the impression that an ecstatic artist had rung out every color of the rainbow, combined them with an insatiable measure of rapturous enthusiasm, and designed the final masterpiece into a fabric that magically protected the wearer from all harm and sadness. What an irony it was that a people with such a sad history, and such a bleak future, could look so perpetually cheerful.

I was later to learn that this area was a shopping Mecca, hundreds of Iraqis flocking there to buy a unique item of clothing that couldn't be obtained in the south. Apparently goods were smuggled in and sold in this region, attracting buyers from all over the country. The city of Sulaymaniyah was built on many small hills in a valley at the bottom of the great Azmar mountains. Out of a population of over one hundred thousand, around nine-eight percent were Kurds with an infamous history. In 1932, during a massive demonstration protesting the election of a new parliament which was to ratify the Anglo-Iraqi treaty of 1930, soldiers had fired on the crowd injuring more than two hundred people and killing forty-five. In June 1963, during the war with the present Ba'ath regime, one hundred and twenty-eight people were rounded up at night and transferred to the outskirts of the city where they were executed en masse and dumped into a huge grave. As bulldozers filled the grave, many were still alive.

It was a city of unfinished projects: the tobacco administration building, the trade unions building, and the sugar factory. Somehow people knew that the war would be starting again, but this was a city where people refused to be silenced. Book stores stocked titles of revolutionary literature that was banned by the government. Back in central Iraq I didn't feel I could speak openly even among friends, and yet here people spoke their minds without apparent fear of reprisal. Their delusion of security came from the March, 1970, agreement between the Ba'ath regime in Baghdad and the Kurdish Movement, which gave full autonomy and self-rule to the Kurds for four years. Gradually, however, even the people who were openly speaking their mind were beginning to see the writing on the wall. This Agreement had been a tactical move by the Ba'ath regime for their own self-preservation.

Although the Agreement had technically been in place for nearly four years, it remained unimplemented; that is to say there had been no true recognition of the Kurdish people as free and equal with the Arab people in Iraq. The most fundamental promise of the Agreement, an official survey delineating the boundaries of one united autonomous region for Iraqi Kurdistan, had not been carried out. Furthermore, the regime resorted to large scale illegal measures to change the composition of some parts of Kurdistan by uprooting large numbers of Kurdish families from their homes and settling non Kurdish families in their houses. Such practices were particularly prevalent in the areas of Khanaqin, Sinjar and the oil rich province of Kirkuk.

On all social, educational, and economic levels, racially discriminatory policies continued to be practiced against the Kurdish

16

citizens, barring Kurdish applicants from enrolling at military and police academies, not appointing Kurds to public offices, and the allocation of medical and social services in the region was virtually non-existent. Perhaps this explains why my presence was so warmly welcomed. Nonetheless, at this point in its history, the city of Sulaymaniyah was controlled by the Kurdish Movement. While there was a strong military garrison and a large active secret service, it was nothing compared with what existed in other parts of Iraq. Most of the local officials were Kurds, including the governor and the police chief. On a very local basis it was in fact the local Kurdish government that ruled, not the central Party.

I quickly became acquainted with these people, making many friends including several doctors who would join the Movement when the war started a year later. One of the most important of these for me was Kurdo. We were introduced through a Kurdish doctor friend of mine, whose brother had been a lieutenant in the Iraqi army. Both the brother and Kurdo had decided to desert at the same time. When I was first introduced to him, Kurdo was disguised as a peasant and hiding out with his family in Sul. He understood only too well the fate that would befall him if his treachery was discovered. He was also painfully aware that the treaty of 1970 was about to fall apart, inevitably leading to the outbreak of war. As a Kurd, Kurdo has always been discriminated against in the Iraqi army even though he'd been a relatively high-ranking officer. He was sickened by the state of affairs in our beloved nation, and dreadfully concerned about what the coming months would bring forth. He was certainly in no way a coward, but equally he was determined he would not be forced to fight against his own brethren in a blood battle that would cost countless lives on both sides. His quick wit and passion for his people endeared me to Kurdo immediately. Little did I know then how our lives wound intertwine over the coming year.

There was an eerie calm, fueled by the hospitable bouquets of baking bread and brewing tea, during the first year I spent in Sul. I would visit the teahouses and attend movie theaters where films were shown from all over the world. It all gave the illusion of being quite open and democratic, but the films were shown in their original languages with Arab subtitles, and most of the people in the region were illiterate. The television broadcasts weren't any better, only showing propaganda for the Ba'ath regime. It was all a little surreal. The times were tranquil, yet everyone could sense the tempest brewing. This was truly the calm before the storm. To understand this properly it is important to appreciate a little more about the historical background of the Kurds.

In the course of its history, Kurdistan experienced the national political division that was present in 1973 in two stages. The first occurred in 1639, when Kurdistan was occupied by and divided between the Persian and Ottoman empires, against the will of its people and despite agreements to the contrary which had been concluded with both empires. This was the first historically recorded breaking of a promise made to the Kurds, who were the true and original inhabitants of Kurdistan. The rulers in Ankara, Baghdad, Damascus, and Teheran have since justified the breaking of promises made to the Kurds by reference to this historical precedent.

After the destruction of the Ottoman Empire at the end of World War I, Kurdistan was divided a second time. In 1923 the homeland of the Kurds was this time severed between Iraq, Syria and Turkey. The initiator on this occasion was the government of Great Britain. Through forced assimilation different parts of Kurdistan developed separate social, economic, cultural, and political structures. Since the Kurdish people in Iraq were forced to resort to armed struggle for their national and human rights, they have been fighting for autonomy within Iraq. On March 11, 1970, the long struggle culminated in a victory with the help of progressive forces in Iraq and internationally. On that day an agreement for a peaceful solution was signed between the Iraqi government and the leaders of the Kurdish revolution. This agreement recognized the legitimate national rights of Kurds, including autonomy within Iraq. But autonomy cannot be achieved without cooperation from all parties.

The urgent need for democracy in Iraq was voiced by progressive forces and stressed by Taakhi, the organizer of the Kurdish Democratic Party, stating (in December, 1970):

"Every country really desiring progress and the elimination of backwardness must consolidate peace and order, save the majority from the dictatorship of the minority, secure justice and legality, enable the people to express opinion and elect their representatives, fight crime and murderers, replace the policy of repression, violence and terror with democratic institutions which guarantee real order and security on a solid basis. These facts have led the Kurdish Democratic Party and the Kurdish people to oppose anti-democratic methods and to resist any measure which weakens the unity of the people and disturbs peace in the country. Our democratic revolutionary principles guide our efforts to create a real national unity, to put an end to acts of violence and terror, to enable the people and their patriotic forces to enjoy their freedom and rights in an atmosphere free from terror and to prevent the minority from arbitrary dictatorial rule and from exploiting its freedom of action to persecute citizens, rob them of their property and encroach upon their constitutional rights."

The Kurdish students in Europe fully supported these democratic demands, because only under democratic conditions for the whole country could peaceful settlement be achieved. Nonetheless new contacts were being made with reactionary tribal chieftains and other enemies of the Kurdish people. There were many examples of attempts to deprive this race of their native identity. On top of that, instead of carrying out land reform and industrialization in Kurdistan, the Iraqi government was settling Arab peasants in Kurdish districts, forcing the Kurds to migrate.

The proclamation of martial law on April 27th, 1971, in eleven provinces of Turkey met with little surprise from informed circles. The preceding events and the accumulation of a series of unsolved social, economic, cultural, and political issues, had always pointed in this direction. In 1972 it was proclaimed that the great dam at Keban (in Kurdistan) would only provide Turkish populated cities with electricity. Kurds were forced to give up their fields, they were discriminated against in numerous ways, and they were governed by 'special' laws. In short, various Turkish governments treated the Kurds as a colony, bringing about social, cultural, and economic imbalance between Eastern and Western Turkey.

Such bitter hardship across the ages has led to some poignant artistic expression among the Kurds. In 1903 Sheikhmus was born in the Turkish province of Mardin. Orphaned at an early age he traveled through Kurdistan, spending time with renowned Sheikhs, where he became a Mullah. Soon after, however, he became disillusioned with the misery and poverty around him. He gave up his beard and his turban and became fearlessly committed to the patriotic struggle. His principal weapon was his poetry which, under the name of Cegerxwin, he would recite everywhere. This ammunition soon made him famous across all of Kurdistan, and it is easy to see why:

O my Motherland, you are the beloved of the world.
Rich in heavenly gardens, meadows and springs,
Bright, charming and vital, gentle and fair,
Full of sweetness, goodness, and youth.
We understand the poet perfectly, then, when he cries:
Not one drop of water from the springs of my Motherland
Would I give for the water of Zemzem, of Kausar, or the water of life,

Not one splinter of rock from our mountain peaks or from our valley
floors,
Would I give for diamonds, rubies or pearls.
Not a maiden, not a bride, not one Kurdish woman, young or old
Would I give for all the houris and angels of Paradise.

Yet still he felt hunted, like a wolf:

Brother wolves, you are brave like us.
But you are giants, the companions of tigers and lions!
You are our companions in misery.
We cry by day and you howl by night.
Kurds and wolves, we are one, like brothers.
We too, like you, flee through the mountains.
We, like you, suffer heat, cold, fog and dust,
And he who among us is killed dies, like you, without a trial.

Eighteen months after the 1970 peace settlement was signed the Ba'athist leadership was admitting Arabs from other Arab states, granting them Iraqi citizenship, and supplying them with financial support, while banishing Feyli-Kurds from Iraq. The Feyli-Kurds had settled in this area prior even to the founding of the State of Iraq as it then was (during the time of the Ottoman domination). Kurds were rounded up nightly from their homes and from the streets and forced to leave Iraq, expelled into either Iran or Turkey where they were housed in horrendous refugee barracks. Although they made up thirty percent of the population, the medical faculty of the university was comprised of only eight percent Kurds. Their needs on every level were overwhelming, but at least as far as medical care was concerned, I was able to assist – a little.

CHAPTER THREE

I spent around eight months working at the general hospital, while 1974 grew ever closer. Everyone seemed to sense it was going to be a hard year, yet this did nothing to stem the wide scale bribery and corruption. It was not an encouraging state of affairs, but I was determined to be of real help where my help was needed most. Sensing the war was coming, I packed my things in two big cases (most of which were medical books) and took a taxi to the outskirts of the city where a land-rover with a Pesh Merga driver was waiting for me. Not in my wildest imagination could I have anticipated the long and arduous journey ahead of me. In hindsight I often wonder had I known then what I know now, would I have remained in Sul? The answer is consistent, swift and resounding. There is no question about it. My destiny lay with the people I saw as my kin, and whatever challenges the fates saw fit to present me with were issues I would simply have to deal with – and deal with them I did.

For security reasons I had told the hospital officials that I needed to take leave to visit my sick father in Baghdad. Perhaps if I had considered the consequence of this deception I might have handled things differently, for it didn't take long for the officials to realize I had not returned to Baghdad. Consequently my father was regularly 'interrogated' (beaten within an inch of his life) by Ba'athists demanding to know my whereabouts. It's a debt I can never repay. At least he survived the experience, which is more than many can claim. He has since told me that he would often shout back in defiance at his tormentors, "You're the government; you tell me where my son is!"

While my poor father was undergoing this torture unbeknown to me, I began my expedition with the Pesh Merga on a paved highway that wound through the Azmar Mountains to the town of Jwarta. The last thirty-five kilometers of this trek took us across unsealed and muddy surfaces, where I found myself wondering if we would ever reach our final destination. In retrospect, given the circumstances that were to follow, those muddy unsealed surfaces would have seemed positively luxurious. This brave new world I was racing blindly towards represented an endless array of tantalizing encounters for a headstrong and rebellious youth who considered himself a revolutionary. What wisdom the passing of years brings. Sadly it's a wisdom many of my comrades were never to acquire.

In due course we arrived in a quaint little town comprised of a main street, a few small shops, teahouses on both sides of the road, and a splattering of modern government buildings and homes. I paid the driver and began making my way towards the local Pesh Merga headquarters. With blinking innocent eyes I entered an innocuous-looking building to find over thirty Pesh Mergas inside. They were all in their twenties and brimming with optimism (some to the point of arrogance). They were also well armed with automatic weapons, plenty of ammunition, and a bountiful supply of hand grenades.

Two officers had been waiting three days for my arrival, both young Kurds who spoke perfect Arabic. Both had left their government army units – one by donating a pint of blood, and the other by claiming his father was terribly sick. I was glad to have their company, but a little less enthusiastic when I discovered the rest of the journey was going to be on foot. The 'direct' route through the wild and rugged mountains was three hundred kilometers shorter, so apparently taking the 'scenic' route by car wasn't an option.

On foot we left for Galala, with two Pesh Merga assigned as our guides. Up until this point all I'd known about revolutions was what I'd read in books. The reality, as I was quickly to discover, was something else entirely. It was impossible to take my suitcases, so I decided to don some civilian clothes and take whatever I could carry in a small briefcase, thinking I would send for my cases later. Iraq had always been a land of extremes and contradictions for me, but only on continuing this journey did I begin to comprehend the magnitude of its ability to delight one minute, while shocking with terror the next. The countryside had been so picturesque, a colorful contrast of high rugged mountains with snow-covered peaks, dropping to green valleys with an abundance of clear cool water below. As I began zigzagging on the next leg of the trip I couldn't help but notice that while it was winter on the peaks, it was already spring in the valleys. Such beauty all around, and yet we'd only been traveling a few hours when the first indication of war was upon us.

When we found a place to stop for tea we discovered everyone excitedly talking about an aerial bomber that had passed the area just twenty minutes earlier. One of the officers accompanying me dropped his expression.

"If that really was a plane, it proves the government means business," he growled.

Without further comment we continued on towards a village called Kamish, which literally hung from the side of a mountain. The plan was to use that as a jumping point to another village where we would remain overnight. During the subsequent three hours of trekking through the wilderness, it began raining so heavily that my sodden shoes felt like lead weights, and my two kilo briefcase might just as well have been an elephant. Once in a while the others would look back to check I was still with them. I was keeping up as best I could, but the thought of maintaining this pace for another eight days seemed impossible. More than once I considered turning around and heading back, but I refused to be a coward. At least I tried to refuse, but when those ahead of me disappeared out of sight I confess I did begin to panic. I was truly alone in the wilds of outback nowhere, picturing myself being devoured by a rabid starving wolf leaping at me from the undergrowth. I had to keep going – one foot in front of the other – that's it, I could do it. The next mountain wasn't all that far away. Not that far. I could make it.

When I finally did reach my next visible target I was relieved to find my friendly escorts perched under the modest shelter of a tree waiting for me.

"There's not much time," one of the officers said simply. "We'll have to find some mules."

And with that minimalist statement, we were off again. I gazed up to the village above. It looked like a bunch of grapes hanging from a tall tree. Almost on automatic pilot I lit a cigarette, not considering my physical condition or the altitude I was at. It was no sooner between my lips when I started coughing and spluttering – it tasted awful. Disgusted, I tossed it away and soldiered on, unable to move faster than a snail's pace and stopping every fifty meters or so to gasp for air. Too often I was struck by a strong wind, forcing me to cling to the nearest rock or bush just to remain upright. It took me an hour and a half to make it to the top, where I once again found my friends waiting for me. This time they were in front of a mosque, the most conspicuous building in the village. I noticed one of the villagers standing beside them as I headed towards the water well to clean up and take a drink.

"Brother Doctor," the villager said urgently, rushing towards me to shake my hand. "You had a hard time making it. Do you think you can make the rest of the journey without mules? The mules cannot get through because of the snow."

I wanted to say, "I could if it wasn't for the briefcase," but instead I answered, "I can try."

"The road to Safrah is about five hours away," one of the Pesh Merga stated. "It will be getting dark soon, and it's impossible to walk on frozen snow. There's no choice. We'll have to stay here until tomorrow and start again at first light."

The villager agreed, and we were cordially invited to stay the night in his home, which was on the opposite side of the area. Gratefully accepting the invitation, we trudged through narrow muddy pathways as people (most of them children) gathered to study us with immense curiosity.

The women of the house immediately took our shoes and socks to wash them, yet even as we enjoyed their hospitality and a good home-cooked meal, it was quickly apparent that I wasn't going to be allowed to rest for long. Before I'd truly had a chance to acclimatize to my surroundings, an old man holding a piece of cloth to his face over a swollen cheek visited our humble abode.

"Where's the doctor?" he asked in a painful voice.

I stood up to examine him; although it was obvious to everyone he had a problem with one of his teeth.

"This is not an issue I would normally attend to," I explained, thinking that sounded perfectly reasonable.

"You're a doctor, aren't you?" the man cried pitifully.

25

My mistake for not pointing out I wasn't a tooth doctor! Not that this would have made any difference. In areas like this even the dresser pulled teeth. ('Dressers' were a vital part of the medical corps.) But the truth was that I had never extracted a tooth in my life. I tried telling the man that I had no instruments, no anesthetics, and no medicine with me. Besides, one is not supposed to extract an infected tooth. I could see by the look on the officers' faces that they were astonished by my explanation.

"You should go to the village dresser to get some medicine for both the pain and the infection. As soon as the swelling has gone down you can have the tooth extracted," I told him calmly.

"But there isn't any dresser here," he wailed. "I'll have to go either to Jwarta or Mawat for the medicine, and they are both almost seven hours walk from here. Usually we get our teeth pulled in Sul, but even if I walk back to the teahouse and wait there for a car, there are very few cars going there at this time."

I really didn't know what to do, but I knew I had to do something. Suddenly, I thought of the needle holder I had in my briefcase, an instrument used to hold a needle in stitching wounds. It was hardly suitable for tooth extractions, but I seemed to be left with little choice.

"There is something I can try," I began warily. "But the instrument I have is not meant to pull teeth. I must warn you, your tooth may break and cause massive bleeding that we won't be able to stop."

"I don't care if you cut my head off," the man screamed in obvious agony. "Please help me."

On plucking up courage to peer into his mouth I could immediately see that all his teeth were bad. The one causing him trouble was already loose, which at least gave me some level of courage. The two officers held his head from behind, while I firmly grasped the offending incisor with my needle holder, twisted it back and forth, and with a deep breath yanked it free from his aching gums. Everyone in the room seemed to release a collective sigh of relief (not least of which was me) but our joyful triumph could in no way be compared to the elation the poor man felt at being liberated from his decaying and infected fang. This was the first time I discovered that necessity truly is the mother of invention – or if not invention exactly, then improvisation. Over the time that was to come

I was going to have to learn to improvise in ways that I wouldn't have believed possible.

The man remained with us until very late, as if nothing had happened. He was even smoking again within half an hour. Marveling at his capacity to recover I decided to clean up, thinking I could then settle in for a peaceful night's rest. I had hardly had a chance to wash my hands when it seemed that everyone with an ailment for miles around had heard a doctor was in town. That night I was flooded with requests for aid, most of them from mothers with sick children. One child in particular I remember had pneumonia with early signs of heart failure. All I was able to do in that case was write a prescription and tell them to get the medicine as soon as possible. I don't know whether they ever received it or not – somehow I suspect not.

By the following morning I was stiff as a board. I couldn't move my legs. My whole body ached. Wallowing in self-pity I massaged my painful extremities before attempting to move. That accomplished, I stood up and instantly realized how shallow caring about my own pain had been. The frail child with pneumonia was still with us, lying motionless and pale only feet away. Gently I examined him again, mournfully reaching the conclusion it was unlikely he would make it through the day. It was heartbreaking, but there was nothing I could do. My medicines were far away, and I was told we had to move on. All I could do was pray.

There was a bitter wind blowing against us that morning, as if in rebuke for my self-pity, or perhaps in retribution for leaving a dying child behind. How little I knew then about the sheer volume of tragic deaths I was yet to witness. They say the first one is always the hardest. That might be true, but now my eyes and my soul have witnessed suffering on a scale my mind could never truly absorb, I can assure it's never easy to see life snatched away from a fellow human being.

The road ahead had not been cleared as few people had attempted to use it. During the winter months these villages were completely cut off from each other, and consequently the outside world. To travel anywhere the men would get together (in some cases as many as eighty) and walk the road, marking it through the frozen snow. My

27

start was very slow, even slower than the day before, if that was possible. I slipped with every step I took, pondering the wisdom of my decision to be part of this crusade. After an hour I couldn't go any further. With all the good will in the world, I had to rest while the others continued. I only stopped for ten minutes, the balance between sheer exhaustion and fear of losing my comrades having become a fine line. When I caught up with the Pesh Merga again one of the officers turned to me, looking down at my feet with a scowl.

"Your shoes are not suitable for this type of weather and landscape."

I conceded the point but asked what I could do about it.

He surprised me by laughing. "Here try mine."

"But what about you?" I gasped.

"I have a spare pair," he said, as though I should have realized that fact.

With sincere gratitude I accepted his army boots and threw my leather shoes away. It was heaven. I felt like a new person. This time I had no trouble keeping up – much to my companions' surprise. One of the Pesh Mergas even offered to carry my briefcase. With that weight lifted from me and my new footwear I positively felt as though I could fly! The rain had stopped, the sun was shining – it was as though we'd slipped into another dimension! Suddenly the scenery was beautiful again; a cacophony of long valleys and high wild mountains alive with beautiful birds of every species. Multitudinous waterfalls welcomed us with streams of clear, ice cold drinking water. There were even a few rabbits hopping around the landscape. For a brief moment it was possible to forget where we were, why we were there, and the inevitable horrors that awaited us.

Around noon we heard the signs of civilization again. The sound of barking dogs told us we were getting close to the village of Safra, an extraordinary feat of engineering that saw the entire village built underground so the roofs of the houses were at street level. From a distance the village was virtually invisible. Access into a home was across the roof and via descent on a flight of stairs. A stranger in this land could reasonably assume people who went to such lengths to disguise themselves would be inhospitable, but nothing could be further from the truth. They welcomed us like long lost family. It was in fact a time-honored tradition in Iraq to welcome strangers, especially among the country folk. No one would refuse entry to a guest, no matter who he might turn out to be.

After lunch we were off to Kanoo, this time with the added benefit of a couple of mules. With Iran just behind the next mountain range we were faced with the options of a treacherous voyage through a wild river or climbing across an ever-narrowing mountain path covered with ice and snow. We chose the latter, despite the fact that even my expert friends had difficulty where the path narrowed in places to around two feet. The flooded river below was being whipped into a frenzy by fierce winds, creating an image of wanting – wanting us to slip and plummet to a watery grave. The faithful mules sensed our nervous tension; it would have been impossible for them not to. Whenever I looked down I felt dizzy, needing to stop for a moment to gather my senses. An illusion of slow-motion pictures zoomed in and out as I gradually began to realize I needn't worry about falling to a watery grave – if I fell I would surely be impaled first on the needle-sharp rocks that paved the way down the mountain to the raging river below.

When finally I noticed the faintest whisper of billowing smoke up ahead I felt the relief of a man stumbling across an oasis in the desert. A small building in the distance was the source of this delight. It was almost out of a fantasy fairy tale – high frozen mountains one minute, and a quaint little building adjacent to a ferry the next. I think the sheer pleasure of knowing I could take a break made my legs buckle beneath me. Muscles I didn't even know I possessed were aching. As I paused momentarily to rub my tender calves, I couldn't help thinking that everything around me was a little surreal. At first I didn't even notice a small village around the little building with welcoming smoke.

The entire township was built right into the side of the mountain on an angle of ninety degrees. How anyone could choose to live in such a place, never mind find the engineering skills necessary to build edifices capable of providing shelter in such a location, was a complete mystery to me. The answer, of course, was several fold. First, such locations were hard for enemy forces to conquer. Second, they always had fresh water. And third, mountain goats thrived in this terrain. It all made good sense, but even so I found myself wondering where the children would play. Then I remembered, the children of these people would have little time, and probably less motivation to play. I was too tired and too hungry to think further.

We tied our mules and headed towards the warm fire in the local teahouse where we found modest sustenance before the time came to leave on the ferry. In modern times the ferry would look like a potential deathtrap, fixed by two cables that ran across a third to pull it over the river without being carried away by the surging currents. The mules flatly refused to embark, despite using every form of persuasion we could think of. The old adage is right, 'stubborn as a mule'. In the end it was decided to tie them to the ferry and let them swim. I felt terribly sorry for them. The river was swollen with icy melted snow, and the current gushed by with disturbing force. Nonetheless, the mules seemed to travel incredibly well under the circumstances. Indeed they seemed happier swimming than bobbing around on the surface of a violently jolting ferry.

Once on the other side we soon approached a cylindrical looking mountain that would be the final stage in our journey to Kanoo. Again the path was narrow and covered in ice and snow, with a whisking wind wishing to whip us to our deaths below. I asked Mustafa, one of our guides, if this would be the last such mountain we would have to climb before reaching our final destination. That was a mistake. In my ignorance I could have believed this would be the last mountain to climb, instead I was informed impassively that there would be another two days of clambering precipices. At that point I completely lost what little sense of humor I had left.

Then it rained – again. Having descended yet another monument, we were forced once again to trudge through mud as a heavy deluge soaked us to our bones. The sight of Kanoo in the distance was a blessed vision indeed. The village was well organized, with large cultivated fields, but the talk around town was clear – the war was about to start again.

We dried off, had a simple meal, and tried to get some rest. The rain continued through the night and was still pouring when my stiff bones were woken at six the following morning. I thought I'd try riding one of the mules this time around, but quickly I discovered being on top of a mule only made me colder, so reluctantly I opted to continue the rest of the way on foot. Yet another village welcomed us during this phase, where we were advised to remain as the continuing rain was making the road ahead impassable. With all due respect to the advice given, we were in a hurry by this point, so regardless of the warning we decided to push on.

Just as we were heading off a small child was brought to me. He was around three-years old and seemed to be suffering from pneumonia with impending heart failure. I couldn't do anything useful except tell the parents how to care for him. I promised to send some medicine back from Qalat Dizah, knowing there would be people there who would be coming back this way. However, I doubted the child would last that long. His liver was enlarged and his breathing difficult; his mother was clearly aware of the reality of his fate. The poor woman was in tears, but infuriatingly there was once again little more I could do than offer her my prayers.

For many more hours we trudged through muddy tracks as the rain continued, leaving us with the impression that heaven was an infinite abyss of tears attempting to drain every last drop from its eyes. After an eternity of traipsing through the full fury of Mother Nature we came at last to a flat area from where we could see Qalat Dizah ahead. It seemed like good news, the only problem was between us and Qalat Dizah was a sea of mud. We literally had to swim through it. With each step I took I sunk, sometimes waist deep, sometimes all the way up to my chest. My shoes were sucked off with each stride. Finally I decided it would be easier to walk barefoot. The poor mules were also having a difficult time. Even though they were strong, every so often they would get stuck and require lifting out of their halter to continue.

Mud-caked and ragged we stumbled into Qalat Dizah to discover a town crowded with people who had gathered from all over Kurdistan. The government army had left a few days before, meaning the area was now under the Movement's control. The shops were still open, and the cafés and restaurants were full of people. Loud Kurdish music blared as we noticed a group of women heading towards the high school building for a meeting. From what I could tell it seemed to be a happy place. Ali, one of my companions, had family there who were prepared to host our accommodations for the night. I was somewhat astonished to find a large brick house with electricity. I hadn't seen electricity for over a week. We were given fresh pajamas, our clothes were washed, and a large meal was prepared. I paid the owner of the mules, who promptly left on his way, so from here on a new method of transport would be required.

We were able to hire a land-rover to take us to the village of Sanga-Cer. It was only one hour's drive away, but it was perhaps the wildest area in Kurdistan. This was considered the front post. It overlooked the Dolly Schahidan – The Valley of the Immortals. With all the mud around, we weren't long out of the village when the land-rover became bogged. It was back to foot trudging. At least there was only one more village before our final destination of Galala.

More hills. More valleys. More mud. And when we reached Sanga-Cer no one was willing to rent us mules to go any further. Thankfully Mustafa wouldn't take no for an answer. He negotiated and bargained, while we shared yogurt, bread and black tea, until it was agreed that one mule owner would travel with us and the mules so long as we agreed not to ride them. At around noon we headed off again, eager to clear through Dolly Schahidan before sunset.

Before long we were faced with another river. It was only around forty meters wide, but it was very deep and very rough, with an L-shaped angle along a rocky hill to our right. The hill was almost perpendicular, looking like a fortress wall. The others decided to climb it, but I knew if I fell from the narrow path I'd be lost because I couldn't swim. Instead it was agreed I would ride one of the mules across. The owner agreed so long as I did nothing to disturb the animal, I was only allowed to hold on tight. The owner crossed via the hill, then called to the mule, once I was astride, to swim across. Red angry water gushed past us, taking the mule by surprise and sweeping us instantly thirty to forty feet off course. I held on – and I prayed. If I lost the mule there would have been no rescuing me. Thankfully the mule was strong, and regained its sense of direction quickly. Gratefully I watched as this gracious and noble beast carried me all the way to the other side.

The following six hours were the most memorable of the trip, and probably some of the most wonderful moments of my life. I can still recall every minute of it with exquisite detail. The aromas of the air, the grass and the flowers were so sweet, so fresh – and so free. The crashing thunder of water falling hundreds of feet into rivers below was almost deafening. Only those who have walked through the Valley of the Immortals could truly understand the primeval grandeur of this deeply spiritual place. The virgin beauty of it all was something utterly awe-inspiring, and I could only feel as though I was in the presence of the Divine. Then we came to the bridge...

The mule owner told us the bridge, which was constructed of wood and mud, was holding but unstable. If the water level from the river below increased any further it would be washed away altogether. Thankfully it held for our crossing, whereupon we took a short respite to break bread and enjoy the fresh clear water. Then – another mountain, this time around five thousand feet high. It took us only an hour to reach the top, and from there I stood under a tree, feeling the snow crunching under my feet, looking back at the untamed magnificence of the panorama we'd navigated. But the time for reflection was brief. There was another three hours traveling before we reached our destination that night – a small house run by the Movement.

When we arrived at our next pit stop, I could see the house was already crowded. There must have been forty people inside, most of them soldiers who had deserted the military garrison in the south to join the Movement. The war was coming; there was no doubt of that.

The following morning I felt enthusiastic. Today we should finally reach Galala. The journey would be through the Barzan highlands; without doubt one of the more beautiful parts of Kurdistan. For a moment I paused. Was I really doing this, or was it all a dream? Either way, what was it all for? Well, for you to really understand that you need to know a little more about the rise to power of one of the most brutal and feared men that history has ever produced – Saddam Hussein.

Born of a sheep herding family in 1937, at age ten Hussein moved to Baghdad to live with his uncle, Khayrallah Tulfah. It was Tulfah who first introduced Hussein to politics and instilled in the boy a deep bitterness towards Western imperialism. As soon as he'd finished school, Hussein joined the Ba'ath Party, a socialist political group committed to Arab nationalism. In 1956 he took part in an unsuccessful coup attempt against King Faisal II of Iraq. Two years later a non-Ba'athist group led by General Abdul Karim Qassin overthrew the king. In 1959, Hussein and other Ba'athist supporters tried to assassinate General Karim Qassin. They failed, so Hussein fled to Syria and later Egypt where he briefly studied law.

In 1963, the Ba'ath Party succeeded in assassinating General Karim Qassin. Hussein returned to Iraq and became an interrogator and torturer for the Ba'ath Party. The Party went through various upheavals and Hussein was imprisoned, yet despite this in 1966 he became Secretary General of the Party with the help of his cousin, General Ahmad Hassan al-Bakr. In 1968, Bakr's faction of the Ba'ath Party seized power and Hussein became Deputy Chairman of the Revolutionary Command Council. This put him in charge of internal Iraqi security and gave him the number two position in the Ba'ath Party. By 1973, Hussein was Vice President of Iraq under President Bakr.

Throughout the 1970s, Hussein consolidated his power. He placed many of his own family members and people from his hometown in important positions in the Iraqi government and military. Family and tribal connections are crucial in Iraq, and Hussein used these ties to his advantage throughout his political career. He also utilized criminals to torture and murder people he perceived as threats.

In 1979, President Bakr resigned under pressure from Hussein, who then became President. Immediately after his succession, Hussein called a Ba'ath Party meeting and had all of his opposition systematically murdered. As President, Hussein continued to reinforce his power base by enlarging security forces and employing family members in the government. One 1984 analysis indicated that fifty percent of Iraqis were either employed by the government or military or had a family member who was, which made the population intimately connected to and dominated by Hussein. But this was not the sum of Hussein's strategy for political survival.

Hussein was not above making humiliating concessions if his grip on power depended on it. In 1975, Hussein made major border concessions to Iran in order to end the Shah's backing of the Kurdish rebellion in the north. Then when he ran into trouble with Iran he even sought dialogue with Israel, despite his uncompromising rhetoric against the Jewish State. Needless to say, Israel did not bite! There was ample precedent for Hussein to lose face whenever his survival required it. Nonetheless, horror in Hussein's Iraq took endless forms.

Even after my journey with the Kurdish people ended, in 1987/88, Iraq's Air Force helicopters sprayed scores of Kurdish villages with a combination of chemical weapons, including mustard gas, Saran, and VX, a deadly nerve agent. Scores of thousands of Kurds, most of them women and children, died horrible deaths. Of those who survived, many were left blind or crippled with agonizing lung damage. But most of the Kurds slaughtered in that season of mass murder were not gassed. They were rounded up and gunned down into mass graves. Those victims were mainly men and boys whose bodies have never been discovered.

In one village, near Kirkuk, after the males were taken to be killed, the women and small children were crammed into trucks and taken to a prison. One survivor, Salma Aziz Baban, described the ordeal to journalist Jeffrey Goldberg.

More than two thousand women and children were crammed into a room and given nothing to eat. When someone starved to death, the Iraqi guards demanded that the body be passed to them through a window in the door. Baban's six-year-old son was one of these. He knew he was dying, and started crying a great deal. When he died in his mother's lap she was forced to pass the body outside, screaming and crying the whole time. Soon after she pushed her way to the window to see if her son's body had been taken for burial. What she saw was dogs roaming a field where the dead bodies had been dumped. With sheer horror she witnessed the legs and hands of her son in the mouths of the dogs. She told the reporter she was silent for a moment before completely losing her mind.

Iraq under the reign of Saddam Hussein was horror without end. Amnesty International once listed some thirty different methods of torture inflicted on the people in Iraq. These ranged from burning, to electric shock treatment to rape; dropping live people in large pools

35

of highly concentrated nitric acid where after a short time only a part of the skeleton remained, and even after executing prisoners the bodies were brought to their families and they were forced to pay for the bullets that were used for the execution. The ears and tongues of hundreds maybe thousands of prisoners were cut off totally without anesthesia. While some governments go to great lengths to keep evidence of torture committed in the name of the State silent, Hussein flaunted his tortures, either leaving broken bodies in the street or returning them to their families. Above all else, Hussein has been an unspeakable evil for the people of Iraq. Crushing him and his dictatorship, liberating one of the most cruelly enslaved peoples on earth, was nothing short of a nearly incalculable mercy.

CHAPTER FOUR

And so we reached Galala, a town built in the 1920s as a British supply route to the Soviet Union through Iran. The road was still a major route into Iran, passing through more primal and breathtaking valleys, this time planted with wheat and barley. The road also traveled to the Choman Valley, which was surrounded by mountains reaching as high as twelve thousand feet. We made our entrance to an area crowded with mules, people, and cars. Mud-bricked buildings climbed the side of the mountain as far as the eye could see. The tea shops along the main street were all crammed with men talking loudly, laughing, and playing games. Busy vendors hawked their goods in make-shift stalls filled with everything one could conceivably want to buy. Could war really be coming to such a seemingly carefree and bustling society?

We checked into the only real hotel in town, and from there went to get something to eat. Even after dark the mood was still buoyant and optimistic. For a while I wondered if I'd imagined the tensions I'd left not so far behind. But I did not need to wonder for long.

The following day I met the chief medical officer of the Movement, who was an important central committee Party member. He greeted me warmly, ensuring me that the Movement needed men like me. We had not been talking long when I felt compelled to ask him how negotiations with the government were going.

"Not so good," he replied somberly. "As you probably know, a high delegation went to Baghdad, to make a final attempt with the government. So far nothing has come of it." He shook his head sadly. "No, the situation does not look good. We have again been cheated."

"What do you mean?" I asked.

37

"It looks certain we are going to have war again. You see the Ba'ath regime has used the treaty of 1970 to destroy the Movement from both inside and out. It allied itself with us only to destroy us."

He let the words hang in the air, silently waiting for my response.

"When I was working in Europe," I began slowly, "and we first heard of the treaty we all thought the Ba'ath were not to be trusted. The government signed the agreement just to prevent their own downfall."

"Exactly!" he snapped back. "In the last four years, since the treaty of March was signed, the Ba'aths have tried to assassinate Barzani twice. No census has been carried out to determine the Kurdish area, as agreed upon. Instead thousands of our people have been forcibly deported from their homes. Hundreds of people have been taken into custody for no reason, only to be tortured or killed." He took a slow breath and studied me for a time. "Well," he began again. "Let's talk about your assignment. I need a doctor in the area of Sul and Kirkuk. It's an important area where the Razgari Brigade is stationed. Yet we haven't had a doctor there in fourteen years. Would you be willing to work there?"

"I have come to serve," I assured him. "It doesn't matter where."

"Good," he said thoughtfully. "I'm glad to hear it."

Almost immediately, everything was arranged. I was later to learn that most doctors who joined the Movement had refused to work in these areas because they were simply too dangerous. In fact one important committee member had changed the assignment of his own son, who'd been scheduled to work with me, saying he didn't want his son killed. When I heard that I felt sad – not for myself, but for 'my' people.

As I prepared to leave Galala I came to learn that this area was considered the unofficial capital of Kurdistan. It was not just the headquarters for the Movement; it was a town of hope. Lying in the Barzani region, comprised of around ten thousand inhabitants, whenever a foreign delegation arrived they had to visit Galala to see the Barzani first. Galala had become a symbol, the stronghold of the struggle to free the Iraqi people from the tyranny in Baghdad, and grant to the Kurdish people the autonomy they had so long been promised. Each day more and more people flooded into the area.

38

Families with their mules, horses, overloaded trucks and cars poured in until the place was bursting at its seams. Thousands upon thousands left their homes and their lands to take up residence here until the bitter end – no matter what the cost.

By this point in time the realization was beginning to sink in that the treaty of March 11th, 1970, was nothing less than subterfuge by the Ba'ath government. It was merely a ploy to buy them time to strengthen their powerbase in order to commit fresh atrocities against the Kurdish people. Four years had been given to ratify the agreement. As March 11th, 1974, ticked ever closer a tense buzz filled the air, like the flight of frightened bumble bees that had lost their hive. On March 10th negotiations between the central government and the Movement broke down. On March 11th, 1974, as the Kurdish delegation left the city of Baghdad, the central government made a broadcast over the radio offering the Kurdish people a ludicrous compromise, which did not include the important and oil-rich province of Kirkuk (an integral part of Iraqi Kurdistan). Leaving Kirkuk out of the agreement would be akin to telling the French they couldn't have Paris.

The Kurds were given fifteen days to accept the offer or face all out war. Not only did the Movement reject the offer, but it seemed the feeling of the Iraqi people generally was in sympathy with the Movement. War was now inevitable. This was a fight to the death – of either the Ba'athist regime or the Kurdish people.

The undefendable cities of Sulaymaniyah, Kirkuk, and Arbil were the first to fall under the control of the central government. The exodus of people was beyond imagination, most of them flooding into areas controlled by the Movement (a high percentage of which eventually found their way to Galala). It was estimated in March alone that over one hundred and fifty thousand refugees poured out of the troubled region. Among these were a mere eighty doctors. The Pesh Merga were around fifty thousand strong at the time, every one of them ready to fight to the death. Even the non-Kurdish people of Iraq were hoping the struggle in Kurdistan would be successful, for they too wanted to topple the much hated Ba'athist regime that had turned Iraq into one giant jail.

The medicine in the area was going to have to be sent in by special caravan. Even before I left Galala, a dresser and a pharmaceutical assistant urged me to take them too for they wished to serve the cause. After discussions with health department officials it was agreed. We left together on March 16th. It was still quiet in Galala, but the tense atmosphere was as oppressive as the regime we hoped to oust. At least it wasn't raining! Six of us in total set out on our grisly duty: Omar (the pharmaceutical assistant) Serwan (the dresser) three Pesh Merga, and myself. Did I say it wasn't raining? I spoke too soon! By the time we actually finished packing and left, sure enough the rain had started to tumble from the sky again. Soon we were trudging through narrow muddy paths between hills en route to our stop for the night, Warti. This time, however, I was in good shape. My muscles were relaxed, I was wearing Pesh Merga khaki and I had decent shoes. Even the heavy weapon I was carrying didn't weigh me down – at least not at first.

Many troubling thoughts raced through my mind, none with happy solutions, but I kept such concerns to myself. Hour after hour we trudged onward until we reached a flooded river where the bridge had been washed away. Not even the strongest swimmer would have attempted crossing the violent torrents that rushed before us. The only hope was that another bridge further along would still be intact. After more marching and trudging we found the next bridge. It was intact, but only just. The construction was an elliptic bridge built of tree trunks and branches, covered with mud that had already been eroded from the heavy rains. The Pesh Merga concluded it would hold for a couple of hours. They must have seen I was none too convinced, so one ran across to prove the point – then another – then the third. Omar and Serwan looked at each other, shrugged, and followed suit. That left only me on the wrong side of the river. The knowledge that I couldn't swim made me feel sick, but what choice did I have? The bridge was only about one meter wide and around ten meters long, so I took a deep breath, virtually closed my eyes, and started to run. I'd managed to reach the half way point when I lost my nerve.

Stranded in the middle of a highly unstable bridge I could hear the water roaring past me, sounding as though it was close enough to lap my toes. I felt dizzy to the point where I very nearly lost my balance.

To screams of encouragement from the other side, I realized it was as far back as it was forward, and the only other option was down. I closed my eyes, took a deep breath, opened my eyes again and raced as fast as I could to the other side. When we arrived at the local teahouse in Warti a short time later, I suspect my eyes were still glazed with fear.

Soaked to the bone, we began to dry ourselves in front of the fire, while we ate bread and yogurt, and drank sweet black tea. It didn't take long for word to spread around the village that I was a doctor, and sure enough the regular procession of sick and injured started a parade for my administrations. With my medicines en route by caravan to our final destination, there wasn't a great deal I could do, but I did recommend firmly to headquarters that a doctor come to visit this (and other) villages on at least a weekly basis from hereon.

More mountains, valleys, rivers, heavy rains, and treacherous bridges awaited. I was becoming quite an expert at all this by now. Occasionally we'd catch sight of some of the indigenous wild animals. The wildernesses of Kurdistan were ironically rich with life. It gave me such pleasure to see so many creatures running wild and free: rabbits, pheasants, bears, deer, mountain goats, wild pigs, wolves, foxes, and a huge variety of bird life. Truly this was a land of contradictions: freedom and oppression, beauty and horror, green valleys and raging rivers – and a richly diverse array of life – and death.

As the journey continued it occurred to me that while I was carrying a weapon I'd never actually fired one in my life. There was little doubt that sooner or later I would be put in a position where I would have to, so a little practice was probably prudent. The Pesh Merga had me aim at a rock on top of a hill about eight hundred meters away. Actually, for a novice, I wasn't too bad. That was before my extremities became so cold I don't think I could have hit the side of a barn with a ten foot pole. Climbing ever upward our soggy clothes became frozen solid. Our hands and feet were icicles. Any sign of spring below had long since vanished. After having witnessed lands so rich in beauty and diversity that they could only be considered natural paradises on earth, I found myself wondering how close to hell paradise really was.

When we made it to the village of Raniyah (after many more encounters with mountains, valleys, mud, rain, gushing flooded freezing rivers, and almost losing Omar as he lost his footing down a mountain slope with his weapon strapped to his back) our next challenge awaited. The medicines that were traveling by special caravan had not arrived, and no one had a clue where they were. This fact was made more heart-wrenching when yet another child was brought to me with pneumonia and potential heart-failure. Quickly I was learning this was simply a part of the territory on the road I had decided to travel; before my journey was ended I would live to see many children die.

After four days of unsuccessfully searching for the medicines we had to move on. A group of twenty policemen had joined the Movement and were heading to our next notable stop en route, Surdash, where the Razgari Brigade was headquartered. This was one of the most, if not *the* most, important Brigades in all of Iraqi Kurdistan, as its experience dated back to 1961. It controlled the whole province of Sulaymaniyah, parts of Kirkuk, and their reach stretched all the way to areas surrounding Galala. We spent the night in Surdash, which gave me the opportunity to have a long chat with the commander. He promised to help my hospital on condition that the medical center would not be moved from one area to another without his knowledge. To this I readily agreed, without having the slightest idea what the conditions would be like where I was heading. Before setting off again I collected another dresser, a medical student, and a dentist, all eager to help the cause. At last I was on the way to the village, and the hospital that I was to call home for the following fourteen months.

CHAPTER FIVE

Under the familiar blanket of heavy rain we reached the outskirts of Azad just as dusk was falling. I remember standing there for endless moments of wonder gazing upon a village that seemed to be lost in time. I was still in a trance-like state when a man who was to become the beating heart of my new hospital came hurrying to meet me with an umbrella. Diman was a courageous and well-trained dresser who had been with the Movement since its conception in 1961. At the age of thirty he'd been assigned as head of the medical corps before my appointment. In my innocence it seemed incredible that a dresser could have been chief medical officer, but at that time I was unaware that no other doctor was prepared to serve in Azad.

Full of optimism and hope, I followed this brave young man to his home noticing all the houses in the village were constructed from mud bricks. Every four or five layers of these bricks were supported by thick planks of wood, and each one was almost identical. Most had only one or two rooms, each with a very small window. I guessed the lack of ventilation and vision was a design specification to insulate the inhabitants from the brutally cold winters in an area where there was precious little firewood.

Most of the houses had fairly large backyards where livestock including cows, mules, sheep, and chicken were kept. It wasn't entirely unusual for these animals to be stabled in the house itself. I found it quite remarkable to see how people with so little could care for their animals so deeply. I supposed on the one hand they did depend on their animals for subsistence; nevertheless there were others in the world who depended on their animals for both their lives and livelihood who did not care for God's creatures nearly so well.

Diman's home was warm and welcoming. A fire was raging in the hearth and the guest room had been neatly prepared. He even had the forethought to prepare fresh clothes for me, which was just as well because mine were muddy and wet through and I was already developing a slight chill. I hadn't taken a bath in two weeks. Momentarily I mused over how quickly I'd come to value as luxuries the commodities I'd grown up taking for granted. What bliss it was to feel the warm water of a bath!

Once I was suitably scrubbed and changed I took a closer look around Diman's home. A typical Kurdish stove took pride of place, a device never seen in the Arabic areas of Iraq. It was a cylindrical shaped barrel around sixty centimeters high and thirty centimeters in diameter. They usually stood on four small legs with a door-like opening for the food. A small narrow flue reached from the oven to the ceiling and extended above the roof. In peacetime these stoves had been made from tin, but during the war four gallon benzene cans provided an effective substitute.

I reveled in a really good home-cooked meal. With a full belly, clean body, fresh clothes, and warm bed I slept well, even though a rather large cat was jumping around on my bed all night. Diman explained the following morning that the cat was there to prevent mice running all over me. Once I understood this the cat certainly seemed the better choice of bedfellows.

Early the next day I was eager to see my new hospital, eager and curious. At first I could not fathom why this place had been chosen as the supposed 'ideal location'. For one thing, it didn't seem near enough to the front. I hadn't yet absorbed that distance and endurance had a totally different meaning to these people from anything I could comprehend. Looking at it from another perspective, the location was ideal. The mountain peaks seemed to touch the sky, creating a naturally fortified citadel. Serwan, who had worked in this area for two years when he was just seventeen, told me that fighter planes could only bomb from one side, and even then it would be impossible because there wasn't enough room to maneuver without colliding into another mountain. Actually this wasn't true, but I was happy to believe it until proven wrong, which didn't take long.

The Susei garrison was a mere twelve kilometers away, and once they started bombing they didn't stop until they lost interest. Heavy artillery shells would hit our village, often four times a week. Usually they would start under cover of darkness and continue until dawn. Amazingly they rarely caused any serious damage, as the surrounding mountains were under Pesh Merga control making any precise targeting by the government forces virtually impossible. I suspect the main aim of these attacks was to wake sleeping children and make the villagers nervous. Militarily speaking their effect was less than impressive. Their bombs often stuck in the snow and mud, the most destructive thing about them being when they finally detonated with stone splinters from the ground. In the summer, when their assaults had the potential to cause more serious damage, most of the inhabitants would leave so the bombs were falling on empty houses.

My first experience at being bombed was when I was busy digging the ground at the bottom of a hill to prepare the foundations for a hospital ward. I remember hearing a horrendous whining sound whiz over us. For an instant I didn't realize what it was. It was only when I looked around to those who were helping me, and noticed they'd all stopped working and were sitting on the ground with stony expressions on their faces, that reality dawned. Then I heard the explosions. I thought I was ready. I'd told myself what it was going to be like. I could handle it. I was there to do a job, and nothing else should matter. But there was nothing that could prepare a person for the cruel, harsh reality of another human being hell bent on blasting you off the face of the earth. The reverberation of the explosion, the shattered shards that flew indiscriminately towards any convenient flesh to imbed themselves in, the looks of resigned horror on what were once innocent faces – nothing can truly prepare anyone for the reality of that.

The winters were bitter, and wood was scarce as the Movement had strict laws about cutting down trees. In fact on one occasion (after the hospital had been established) I was called into the Revolutionary Court because my people at the hospital had cut down too many trees and the owner of the land had complained to the judge. Luckily the judge was a good friend of mine, and I explained I had twenty-three stoves to heat in the hospital to keep everyone alive. We tried explaining to the landowner that the wood was to save wounded people, but some people on this earth are only interested in themselves. Luckily the judge wasn't one of them. He told the landowner in short order that he was 'anti-revolutionary' and threw the case out of court. I was sad that so many trees were destroyed during the winter months, but there was no other source of fuel. Petroleum (which would have sufficed) was hard to come by and invariably under central government control.

My entire journey up to this point had been with one goal in mind – to get a hospital established to treat the needy. When at last I was introduced to the building that had been earmarked for this purpose I couldn't believe my eyes. The windows were broken, the front door was almost falling off, and I learned after the March 1970 agreement it had been used as a stable! As I began my inspection a big crowd gathered to stare. Omar and Serwan were by my side. Although neither ever looked surprised at anything, they didn't look overly impressed either. There was nothing for it but to step inside and see what wonders awaited us…

Oh, the smell! The rooms were covered with animal dung that must have been piled a foot high. The mist of rotting excrement was like ringing a dinner bell to indigenous disease carrying rodents, many of whom I could see darting in and out of their hidey holes.

"How can I set up a hospital in such an unsanitary place?" I wanted to know.

I must have wondered out loud if the building had been chosen because it was at least safe from artillery shells, but this prospect was soon quashed too.

"Where raindrops fall, shells can fall," a villager told me matter-of-factly.

If I had wanted a challenge – I had one!

Later that same day I met two people who were to become two of my closest and most trusted friends. The first was Ali, a local Pesh Merga who hadn't seen much action, and consequently had been assigned to the medical corps as a cook (although I soon had to relieve him and treat him for tuberculosis). The other was Bahnaz, who was a medical technician from the city of Sul. Bahnaz was one of those people who was good at just about everything, and as an added bonus he'd managed to bring with him plenty of medical supplies, furniture, and what turned out to be one of the most important ingredients in our little gulag – hundreds of kilos of DDT. After a cup of particularly strong tea, I gathered my forces and commenced the cleaning campaign.

While one group dug dung, another cleaned ceilings, and a third began the job of stuffing hundreds of rat holes with DDT. Altogether we removed nearly two tons of animal excrement! The entire building needed to be sprayed inside and out, not only because of the rats but also to keep out snakes, scorpions, and malaria carrying mosquitoes. It was frontier heaven – or was that hell? I knew all that DDT wasn't going to do my patients much good, but there was no other option. We'd just have to let the building dry and air before it could be open for business. Clearly it was time to take a tea break.

The teahouse was full of people, well to be more precise it was full of men, as it was against custom to allow women in. Kurdish music was blaring loudly as games were played and conversation buzzed. I didn't think anyone would even notice we were there, yet I was no sooner through the door when everyone seemed to want to shake my hand. It was an extremely humbling experience.

As days passed the hospital became an important center for the hundreds of people visiting Azad daily. Many new cafés were opened to accommodate the influx of trade, and as I recall two new restaurants were even established. Almost everyone who came to town was suffering either from an ailment or injury, and most of those were Pesh Merga. Only the serious cases were admitted to hospital, the others were appropriately treated and either sent back to their unit or advised to rest up in the village for a few days. Accommodating 'out patients' in such a fashion was never a problem. Villagers were only too happy to open their homes and their hearts to strangers in need, especially if those strangers were Pesh Merga. It made no difference how poor or wealthy the villager might be; their generosity of spirit was the same. Whatever these villagers had they were prepared to share. If only all in the world held this attitude the planet might be a much kinder place to live.

I wish I was able to express my true feelings of admiration and love for these people, but no words could ever suffice. When I look back on it now, although I lived with them for fourteen months, I still feel I hardly know them at all. The village was composed of only one hundred and fifty families, who largely came from three identifiable tribes. There was a little friendly rivalry between the tribes, but that was all it ever amounted to. At one point in history the village had been owned by the grandson of perhaps the most popular Kurdish leader of modern times, Sheik Mohmoud, a man who had led the most important Kurdish uprising against the British between 1919 and 1930. In the mid 60s, his grandson turned against the Movement, and the Movement consequently declared the land a liberated area. The territory was divided equally between the three tribes, the native villagers using the land to plant vegetables, tobacco, grain, barley, and grapes. The most important of these crops by far were the grapes. All the surrounding hills were covered in huge vineyards, the produce from which was sold in the markets of larger towns and cities. However, since the war flared up again no one was permitted to travel to the markets, which meant there was no shortage of grapes to eat!

The farmers were simple people, who never demonstrated any desire to improve their standard of living. They only wanted to be free to live the way they had chosen to live. They were never really actively involved in the fighting, although the first Pesh Merga killed in the conflict of 1961 was from this area (in fact there was an outfit named after him). The busy main street remained active despite the war, and somehow they managed to keep constant supplies of soap, toothpaste, cigarettes, matches, tea, sugar, rice, and several other basic necessities. There was also a good deal of skilled labor, including a blacksmith who was invaluable to us in building the hospital.

The main street divided the village into two halves. One of these was largely composed of orchards (brimming with both fruit trees and tall bamboo-like trees). Countless streams trickled their way through this half of the area, winding their way past the mosque that sat proudly in the center of town. This edifice was well hidden among tall leafy trees, but nonetheless in 1967 a Mig 19 managed to hit it directly with two rockets. In 1974 the two large holes left by the attack were still quite evident.

48

With hard work and dedication these people helped me finish preparations for my hospital. The broken windows were covered with clear plastic, the ceilings with yellow plastic, and the walls with green plastic. The plastic made cleaning easier, as well as affording effective protection from the assorted wildlife that might have wished to return to their former home. The building was divided into four areas: an examination room, a dressing and injection room, a pharmacy, and living quarters. The pharmaceutical area seemed to stubbornly remain moist, so it was necessary to put a large stove in there to keep it dry. We had plenty of lab equipment, a medical balance with weights, large bottles (called Winchesters) that were used to store pharmaceutical mixtures, and an ESR apparatus. This device was helpful in indicating the presence of a serious internal infection, which was particularly useful when it came to diagnosing the ever-present tuberculosis as there was no X-ray equipment.

Omar proved to be a skilled pharmaceutical assistant, so things were looking reasonable except for one important element – we had a woefully low supply of medicine. We had trunks, chairs, tables, shelves, and even an examination table, but the medicines that had gone missing from Galala were still unaccounted for. In theory the delivery should have arrived before I did, but the heavy rains that led to the destruction of many bridges delayed this well-thought out plan. Despite this troubling setback we ploughed on cleaning and organizing our new facility until it came close to resembling something like a hygienic and functional public utility. All too soon we were open for business.

I was having dinner one evening when someone told me a very sick girl had been taken to the hospital. Her parents had brought her from Sargelow, a three-hour walk away. When I heard that, I immediately gave instructions for the stoves in my examination room to be heated up, that at least two lamps should be lit, and I hurriedly headed off to attend my patient. She was a pretty blonde girl around six years old, but I could immediately see her condition was serious.

"Please, brother doctor," her mother implored, "save her! She is the third of my children who would die this year."

Through her weeping she told me there were another two children at home who were also ailing, but it was impossible to bring them all on the arduous journey necessary to reach my hospital. Her husband tried to calm her, but the poor mother just kept on weeping. I attempted to get a handle on how the condition came about by asking questions while rectally taking the girl's temperature. It read 39.7 degrees centigrade – far too high. The first priority was to get that temperature down. Cold compresses were immediately ordered while I continued to try and get the case history from the mother. I had learned from past experience that getting medical case history from a parent was a less than reliable source of information. Aside from the emotional trauma of dealing with a sick child, and not knowing what to look for in terms of symptoms, these people were in the middle of a war and hence preoccupied with keeping themselves alive – recording medical case history as minor symptoms began to appear was hardly a priority.

After much prompting I managed to ascertain that this particular little girl fell sick around eight days earlier. The early signs had been severe diarrhea, vomiting, and for the last two days there had been fever, convulsive seizures, and urinary retention. The child refused all fluids and until this day had been restless and crying continuously. It was no surprise then that at this point she was unconscious with at least five percent fluid depletion, her breathing was hard, her pulse was rapid, her blood pressure was low, and her abdomen was rigid. As I examined her a fresh mild convulsive attack took place, and I could also see her liver was enlarged. These signs suggested I look for meningitis. The convulsions could have been caused by the continuous high fever, but this didn't account for the rigidness in her neck. Even the position she was lying in suggested meningitis. The abdominal rigidity was due to the urine retention, but the question was, what caused the retention? Whatever the diagnosis it was plain to see the condition was serious, and swift action was required if there was to be a chance of saving the child.

I asked my new right-hand man, Diman, to boil a thick long needle and prepare the largest syringe we had. He headed off into the dressing room and returned a short while later with a 10 cc syringe and a normal sized needle (which was the largest we had). We boiled the needle along with an artery in a kidney-shaped bowl. While waiting for the instruments to be sterilized, I asked Diman if there was a scale anywhere. The only thing he could think of was a small flat scale in his home. It would have to do. Ali was instantly dispatched to retrieve it, and ten minutes later everything was ready. I'd never conducted a bladder puncture on a small child, and in truth the needle was too small for the job. Customarily such administrations were not practiced, as to push a bladder catheter through the vagina could cause loss of virginity. However, this was hardly my primary consideration at that moment. I disinfected the lower abdomen with alcohol, and dug deep inside myself to search out a level of confidence. The parents were asked to wait outside, which happily they agreed to without objection (as it was also not customary for a male doctor to attend a female patient).

I put the needle on the syringe. We had no local anesthetic but the unconscious girl wasn't feeling anything – thankfully. If I was successful it would be of great relief and prevent further kidney complications. I pushed the needle through the skin in the middle line with a forty-five degree angle with the bowel skin and at once, without even pulling on the syringe handle, the syringe was filled with deep yellow urine. The tension in the room was palpable. I told Diman to fix the needle with the artery just above the skin and keep it tight while I emptied the syringe. Over the next ten minutes I withdrew around 400 ml of urine. When the parents rejoined us and saw the quantity of urine that had been extracted they looked quite relieved. The next step was for me to weigh the child. For this to occur I asked the father to step on Diman's scales, then step off, pick up his daughter, and step back on. The difference between the two weights would hence represent the child's reading.

The mother was instructed to give her daughter glucose water that we'd prepared until morning – over half a liter of it. The patient withstood the initial injections very well, but she was still having difficulty drinking. As the night unfolded this situation improved. Over the next hour and a half we managed to bring her temperature down with the aid of cold compresses and aspirin. It was now reading 38.6. It wasn't ideal, but it was hopeful, and at that point that's all we could do – hope. Ali brought the parents some fresh tea and bread, and in the next room we all kept a round the clock vigil in case my small patient was in need of further services through the night.

Almost all the medicine available in Kurdistan amounted to penicillin and aspirin, and there were only so many ways a doctor could get creative with these drugs, but it was better than nothing.

As we drank tea one of my medical students, Adil, asked about my diagnosis. I explained it was difficult to point to a single diagnosis in these circumstances, but in turn asked my student if he had recognized the clinical symptoms of fluid loss. He was a smart man.

"The dry tongue, the fever, the hollow sunken eyes, the dry feather-like skin, the muscular weakness, and the distended abdomen," he replied correctly. "But why did you give her the heart drug, digoxin?"

"The child is also suffering from acute heart failure," I explained. "This was evidenced by the hard breathing, the rapid pulse, and the enlarged liver. The heart trouble was caused by the fluid depletion – the pneumonia was just an additional complication." I paused before voicing the deepest of my concerns. "I think the girl is suffering from meningitis – you saw the neck rigidity, the convulsions, and the typical hunting dog's position?"

Adil nodded sadly.

A short while later the girl's mother started shouting. We all ran into the examination room where the poor woman was going quite insane, not only screaming but actually pulling her hair. The reason for her grief was obvious. The child had started convulsing again. I told Diman to get the mother outside, while I grabbed the syringe that was still on boiling water. Using a third ampoule of sedative I injected her quickly. It took a few minutes, but the convulsions stopped and happily her temperature was now down to 38 degrees. Despite the horrendous condition of this poor child, I was feeling quietly optimistic. Even though she was under heavy sedation her breathing was good again, and her pulse was almost normal. I'd have given anything for a lumbar-puncture needle to reduce the liquid pressure in the spinal cord, but that was not to be. Once the convulsions stopped I called the mother back in, assured I would do everything within my power to save her child, and instructed her to continue giving as much sugar water as possible.

At two in the morning I gave the child a second shot of penicillin. Her temperature was stable at thirty-eight degrees. The good news was the girl had regained consciousness and was sitting up. Diman and Adil were utterly exhausted, so I sent them home. Bahnaz had been with me the entire time, and he wasn't going anywhere. He offered to stay awake and take care of whatever was necessary, an offer I gladly accepted with the proviso he woke me up if I was needed for anything. I had no intention of leaving the hospital; I just needed to grab a few moments sleep.

By 7am I awoke to see Ali making tea. He'd also heated some water for me to bathe in. I peaked outside. It was raining – naturally. I only hoped the climate was sunnier in my examination room. With much anticipation I headed in to inspect my small patient. Her mother looked wrecked, but the small child was awake and had been drinking fluids all night. Her temperature was still 38 degrees, but her abdomen was soft, her heart action and pulse were steady, and her breathing was normal. She was over the critical stage, the drugs were doing their job, and there'd been no complications. I felt sure that one little soul at least was going to be just fine.

A short while later Diman returned with a small covered pot.

"I've brought some fresh home-made yogurt," he smiled. Diman only had one cow left, but she produced plenty of milk so there was no shortage of yogurt. Yogurt, fresh bread and black tea was the best breakfast you could have in Kurdistan, a fact I never got used to. To be honest, I'd rather have gone without breakfast, or at least only had the bread and tea. We gave some of the yogurt to the patient, which she had some difficulty with at first, but soon she was eating quite well. Her loving mother was spent, so when I heard she had relatives in the village I sent her to get some rest while the father remained on hand.

In practical terms we hadn't been ready to open the hospital but as any doctor who has taken the Hippocratic Oath will tell you, it's impossible not to do all that is possible to help a fellow soul in need. While we continued working to get the pharmacy and dressing room ready, whenever villagers appeared wanting assistance they were never turned away. I only prayed that the medicines from Galala would turn up soon.

The first official house-call we made was to a sixty-year-old woman. She was lying at home in a dry room with the window

53

closed. The stove was very hot and there were ten people around her, all of whom stood up when Omar and I arrived. It was customary in these parts for people to stand whenever a stranger entered, and remain standing until the stranger sat down. Instead I asked for them all to leave so I could examine the patient. The son and his wife remained, listening to the painful story that the ailing woman told. She'd had heart trouble for two years but due to the war her son couldn't take her to Sul for treatment any more. Her legs were swollen and she had difficulty breathing. It was quite clear she was suffering from chronic heart failure with high blood pressure. Fortunately this was something I was able to treat as I had enough of the necessary medicines for this condition. I conducted the required administrations, left instructions for her care, and headed to the next patient who was a few doors away.

The second patient was a tiny thirty-nine year-old woman with an advanced case of Pott's disease. There was nothing I could do to alter the progress of the illness. The patient was so weak, and her bone deformations were so well-developed, that she could no longer walk at all. She told me she'd been ill since early childhood, but the condition had progressed over the last six years. Her husband had taken her to many doctors in Sul, but due to the war this was no longer possible. It was with a heavy heart that I advised Diman and Ali this condition was a form of bone tuberculosis; consequently there was little we could do to assist.

The third patient was on the other side of the village, where the tall trees shaded fresh water wells. The son of the patient led us into the yard where we climbed a ladder to the living quarters. Taking our shoes off, we followed him down a hall to the main room. Inside around fifteen people surrounded the patient. Behind them I could see an old man lying beneath the window. I barely needed to examine him to see he was gravely ill, and likely beyond the reach of any medical administrations. Everyone in the room was on their feet, as we were yet to take a seat. Once again I asked them all to leave. Slowly I pulled back the cover over the old man to reveal a body that must have been six feet and eight inches tall, all of it covered with just skin and bone. His abdomen and legs were massively swollen, and he was deathly pale. The son told me his father had been sick for

54

the last six months, but during the past two weeks he hadn't managed to eat or drink a thing. Even when he tried to drink water he'd vomit it up. The son had managed to take the old man to Sul on the 8th of March, three days before the war started, but at that time there were no doctors there.

The father was in his late sixties, and suffering from a malignant tumor. I had no morphine, nor any of its derivatives, indeed no strong pain killers of any sort. I was beginning to feel utterly impotent. Everyone expected the new doctor to save lives – to perform miracles – and all I was able to do was confirm their worst fears. I had no medicines, well none to speak of. I couldn't even ease his suffering. I was a warrior without a weapon, and my heart ached with the weight of this sickening truth. There was, however, one thing I could do – should do – had to do – I had to tell the son the truth.

"Is my father seriously ill?" he asked.

"Very seriously," I assured him. "I'm sorry to tell you but by all the indications your father will not be with us longer than a few days. Even if you could get him to Baghdad, the result would be the same."

The son considered my words somberly for a few moments. "What should I give him to eat?"

"Anything he wants," I told him sadly.

It was another heart-wrenching fact I had to learn to live with. Over the fourteen months I was in Azad I was often confronted with cases I had inadequate medicines to treat. However, there was one ray of sunshine. The small girl who had traveled three hours to be my first in-house patient was improving. She was still drinking and her temperature was almost normal. I decided to keep her in for another night before releasing her into her mother's care. The mother studied her child before turning questioningly towards me.

"Will my child be well now?"

I looked at her and smiled. "With God's help, I hope so."

I glanced towards Diman. He was smiling too. In amongst all this horror, this little ray of sunshine gave us cause to smile. Then I thought about what I'd said… "With God's help." Those words somehow rang in my ears.

I thought of a God I'd never known…

A God who watched while cruelty and injustice raged…

A God who did nothing to stop the brutal, senseless killing of innocent lives...

A God who did nothing to stop the meaningless destruction...

A God who slept while we struggled for our freedom.

CHAPTER SIX

Once the hospital was officially opened for business we were flooded with patients. I hired a villager who could read and write to assign everyone a card with a number. It was also his job to try and ensure that those waiting remained quiet. A further two villagers were hired to keep the place clean. Arriving at eight in the morning, there were already around thirty people waiting to see me, most of them women and children. But this number quickly swelled to over one hundred. It was raining (of course) so everyone had to wait inside, which, needless to say, caused overcrowding and disorder. No one was used to the numbering system, a detail I had to remain quite firm on. In fact I soon devised a system whereby I treated people who had traveled from other villages first, before those local to Azad, to allow them sufficient time to travel home again. Far from objecting, as you might suspect, the locals were proud to wait, believing they were doing their small part to help others. Only the most serious cases were seen as soon as they arrived, no matter where they were from.

On the first day the hospital was officially opened for business I saw ninety-seven people in the morning, and fifty-two in the afternoon. There was still precious little medicine available, but Omar managed to prepare enough mixtures of penicillin and aspirin to last for a week, seeing an average of one hundred and thirty patients a day. The villagers had an interesting way of looking at things. If they were given an injection they were happy, but no one was pleased at the thought of taking tablets (a fact that was also true in the Arabic part of Iraq). It was apparently important for them to feel a stethoscope on their chests, and have their blood pressure taken, so these pieces of my medical equipment were put through their paces on a phenomenal level.

No serious cases came forth on the first day. The most interesting was a young mother with her nine-year-old daughter. The mother had tuberculosis, which she'd been treated for in Sul. However, her treatment had been terminated when her husband, a Pesh Merga, had to leave the city. She showed me her medical card, which indicated she was supposed to be on a daily dose of streptomycin 1g injections, and P.A.S. tablets. Both the woman and her daughter looked very pale. Her left elbow was massively swollen with a big abscess that covered the entire joint area. Movement in her left hip, as well as her elbow joint, was painfully restricted. The abscess needed to be opened, but we still had no anesthesia, and worse still we had no sharp scalpel. All we had was a pair of scissors and a torn pair of surgical gloves. I told Diman to cut as many drains as possible and boil them. We gave the child a sedative injection, and while Serwan prepared the instruments we had to open the abscess. Both patients were going to need to attend the hospital daily; the mother for her injections, and the daughter for separate treatment.

The mother's arm required a splint after the abscess had been opened. Bahnaz was able to obtain some materials to construct a makeshift splint, which comprised simply of wood covered in ordinary cloth as there were no bandages or cotton. Helping people back into good health was testing to say the least in such adverse conditions. There were many cases of acute bronchitis, pneumonia, and chronic diarrhea among the children. Most of them were also suffering from malnutrition. Sadly I also had the misfortune of meeting the fourth case I had witnessed of a marasmic child. I had seen three cases in Sul, and this one was no different. The boy looked like a small monkey, covered only in skin and bone.

"How old is your son?" I asked the mother.

"He is two years old, brother doctor," she told me.

The boy only weighed four and a half kilos. I know a professional is supposed to remain objective from his cases, but it just wasn't possible. The heartache I felt looking at this tiny soul was indescribable. I needed effective drugs, plasma infusions, and more importantly I needed time to teach the mother how to properly care for her infant. All I was able to do, however, was ask the mother to bring her son to me on a daily basis, but it was self-evident there was little I was going to be able to do to save his life.

The majority of women I saw were suffering from anemia, most likely due to multiple pregnancies and malnutrition. They also suffered from back pains due to heavy manual labor and having to carry water from the wells. On top of this it was common to see kidney and urinary tract infection, as well as genital infections.

The little blonde girl I'd treated early on improved well. When I visited her in her relative's home, her father told her to stand up and kiss my hand. The very nervous child reluctantly stood. I could see she was shaky on her feet, so I kissed her forehead and told her to sit down again. It gave me great joy to see how quickly she'd improved, but I urged her parents to remain in Azad for a few more days in order for me to finish her treatment. From there I went to check on my first official house call.

The woman was doing well. Her legs were no longer swollen, and her blood pressure and pulse were fairly stable. The digoxin and lasix had really done the job, but Serwan and I were nonetheless seen as the masters who worked these wonders. Well, that was some good news, so with that positive thought we headed to our next stop, the patient who had Pott's disease.

I was happily surprised to hear the woman tell us she'd tried walking for the first time in six years that morning. She had succeeded in standing up against a wall unaided, which was quite remarkable. Although there was no chance of improving her general condition, the fact that her spirit had been sufficiently lifted to give her a glimmer of hope was heartwarming. Her husband was a rich farmer, who sent us a huge turkey in a gesture of gratitude. With humble thanks we returned the gift, explaining we were here to help the people of the revolution and seeing people responding to our administrations was all the payment we would ever need. This altruistic attitude couldn't prevail for long, however. As the war progressed and conditions deteriorated, we learned not to turn away gifts of food. Our patients needed nourishment, and consequently the gifts were given directly to the hospital cook who would prepare and distribute what was on offer among those in need.

The tall man with the tumor only lasted a few days, as I'd predicted. I couldn't help but think how tragic it was that he would never live to see a free Iraq. From a historical perspective it is probably important here to explain how the Ba'ath Party came to rule the region with such an iron fist...

Both the Syrian and Iraqi Ba'ath Parties originated in the Ba'ath Movement, an Arab political movement which began in the early 20th century. It was founded by Syrian thinkers, most notable Michel Aflaq. Two other major proponents of the early Ba'athist ideology were Zaki al-Arsuzi and Salah al-Din al-Bitar. Like Alfaq these men had careers as middle-class educators, and their political thoughts were influenced by Western education. Many early Ba'athists also professed Christianity. The movement found support among the more republican wing of Iraqi soldiers in the British and later the Hashemite services.

The Ba'athist Arab Socialist Party was officially founded at its first Party congress, held in Damascus, April 7th, 1947. The early Party formed in opposition to both French colonial rule and to the older generation of Syrian Arab nationalists, and advocated instead Pan-Arab unity and Arab nationalism. Its constitution blended non-Marxists socialism and nationalism. The early Syrian Ba'athists opposed the influence of Europe in their country's affairs, and used nationalism and the notion of unifying the Arab world as a platform. Ba'athists always claimed to speak for the entire Arab nation and the progress of the masses, although the Party remained extremely small, factional, and often reliant on nationalist radicals in the militaries. However, its influence quickly spread to other Arab countries by 1954-58, and branches formed in Iraq, Jordan and Lebanon.

Iraqi and Syrian Ba'athism today differ widely and partially oppose each other. They share one common feature in that under Saddam Hussein Iraq also moved away from Ba'athist principles. In Iraq the Ba'ath Party remained a civilian group and lacked strong support within the military. The Party had little impact, and the movement split into several factions after 1958, and again in 1966. It lacked strong popular support, but through the construction of a strong Party apparatus the Party did succeed in gaining power.

The Ba'athists first came to power in the coup of February, 1963, when Abdul Salam Arif became president. Interference from the Syrian Ba'athists, and disputes between the moderates and extremists, culminating in an attempted coup by the latter in November, 1963, served to discredit the extremists. However, the moderates continued to play a major role in the succeeding non-Ba'athist governments. In July, 1968, a bloodless coup brought to power the Ba'athist general, Ahmad Hassan al-Bakr. Squabbles within the Party continued, and the government periodically purged its dissident members. Saddam Hussein eventually succeeded al-Bakr in 1979. Although almost all the Ba'athist leadership had military background, under Hussein the Party changed dramatically and became heavily militarized with his leading members frequently appearing in uniform. This began to occur even while Hussein was 2IC of the movement during the war in which my hospital was built.

The Kurdish situation in Iraq is a complicated and sensitive issue that can only be completely understood through a careful study of Iraqi politics dating back to the origins of this Middle Eastern nation-state. Only after identifying the key elements of Iraq's governmental infrastructure can you comprehensively show the fundamental differences between Iraqi and Kurdish political and social dogma. It is these differences that fostered the epic tensions between two groups and had sown seeds for rebellion within Kurdistan. Throughout history, and primarily after World War I, the Kurdish minority in the Middle East had been effectively used as a political ally only to further another regime's socioeconomic needs. Consequently the Kurds have been traditionally labeled as the perpetual scapegoats of the Middle East. This exploited and often unnoticed people sought only a homeland for their eclectic yet unified nation. Iraqi Kurds were almost completely without a voice in central politics.

As the Ba'ath Party consolidated its powerbase, the Kurds were seen as potentially hostile to the creation of this Arab-orientated philosophy. As a result the Kurds were seen as an obstacle to the goals of the Ba'athist Party. The Kurds lay a historic claim to the land we call Kurdistan, which encompasses sections of south east Turkey, northern Iraq, western Iran, Armenia and north east Syria. As a point of fact, the Kurds have lived in this region dating back to 2400 BC.

Most of Kurdistan, however, was conquered by Arabs in the seventh century and converted to Islam, the region later falling to the Ottoman Turks. From antiquity the Kurds have been proud, tough, and resistant to foreign influence. To this day the Kurds remain distinct from the people of the countries in which they reside. They are known for their ferocious defense of harsh terrain, their almost entirely self-sufficient economy, and their tribal-orientated society. Even today the vast majority of Kurds live in small villages, defying the modern culture that has been embraced elsewhere. In the rural areas the political and social organization is still based on descent, clans, and land ownership. Leadership is divided between the mir or beg, who leads the tribe, and the sheikhs or mullahs, who are the religious leaders.

The Kurdish Democratic Party (KDP) became the collective voice of Kurdish factions after World War I, formed as a reaction to revoked promises of a Kurdish homeland as stipulated in Article 62 of the Treaty of Sevres. Perhaps ironically, Kurdish nationalism became both defined and subjugated after the establishment of the Ba'ath Party in Iraq, inextricably intertwining the Kurdish history with that of Iraq. The ideology of the Ba'ath Party calling for Arab unity stressed a need to overcome artificial boundaries put in the place in the Middle East by colonial powers. In theory the Ba'athist philosophy was open to all inhabitants of the Arab nation, regardless of tribe, religion or ethnic origin. But in reality, the Iraqi adoption of the doctrine proved to be a crushing blow to Kurdish aspirations, and the Ba'ath Party proved to be a means to muster Iraqi aggression against their Kurdish 'brethren' in the north.

By the end of 1969, Saddam Hussein, then vice-chairman of the RCC, began to take a more visible role in Ba'athist politics. Hussein shocked everyone by signing a peace agreement with the Kurdish Democratic Party on March 11th, 1970, despite including the seemingly innocuous resolution for the RCC to wield some influence over economic, legal, and governmental issues within Kurdish borders. The agreement was always destined to fail. Since the creation of modern Iraq, the Iraqi Kurds have been repressed. An aggressive military operation against the Iraqi Kurds was part of an ongoing larger campaign against the Kurd's struggle for autonomy with the Republic of Iraq. The broad purpose of the campaign was to eliminate any resistance by the Kurds by any means. Its specific aim was to 'cleanse' the region of 'saboteurs', who included all males between the ages of 15 and 70. Mass executions were carried out, economic blockades put on villages, and anyone who refused forced relocation was shot. Even when they agreed, the men were often separated from the women and children and shot anyway. It seemed like a hopeless battle, but with my little hospital, as poorly stocked as it was, I was determined to save as many of the brave souls as I possibly could.

In the first two months of my operation in Azad a few events took place that would influence all that happened in the coming year. On the third day after I arrived, the commander of the Ruzgari division came to the village to visit his family. He was a man of modest stature, around fifty-five years of age, and a former major in the army.

"At last," he almost sighed with relief as he spoke to me. "This is the first time since the revolution started in 1961, that a real doctor has come to our area."

Apparently Adil and Diman had spoken well of me. It felt as though I'd already made a good impression on the man before we were formally introduced. I explained we had no medicine, no surgical instruments, and not enough dressers for a hospital servicing the front line of the fighting. On top of that we had no money, and virtually no food supplies. He smiled at me, which I took to be a rather odd reaction.

"As you know, the military budget is separated from the health budget, but since you have volunteered to serve our Brigade, I am willing to loan you some money."

"But I have no idea when I'll be able to pay you back," I complained.

"It doesn't matter," he replied kindly. "The important thing is that the health department will pay it back in time. As far as the medical supplies are concerned, all I can do is to send an urgent telegram to our leadership requesting stock be sent as soon as possible, along with additional dressers." He turned to Diman. "Hire three mules and come here as early as you can tomorrow. I will give you all the supplies and money I can spare."

We spoke little more on that occasion, but as time unfolded we became good friends. Ironically (or perhaps poetically) our friendship was also destined to turn into a doctor/patient relationship over time. I didn't foresee any way of repaying this man's kind loan, but he never mentioned it again.

As though a miracle occurred, or a mirage manifested, it was during this same period that the mysteriously missing medicines from Galala finally showed up. Much of the stock had been damaged or 'lost' along the way, but there was enough to give us the boost we desperately needed. Simultaneously a further two recruits joined the medical corps. One was a young doctor who had been a friend of mine in Sul. The other was a lab technician in his final year of studies who was clever, industrious, and brimming over with enthusiasm.

The doctor from Sul had been sent to help me run the administration of both the Kirkuk and Sulaymaniyah provinces. Although the cities of these areas were under government control, the hundreds of villages and towns in the surrounding areas, populated by hundreds of thousands of people, were still in the Movement's control. He was to be the doctor in charge of the 1st, 2nd, and 3rd battalions of the Ruzgari Brigade operating adjacent to Kirkuk, and I was to take care of the main Brigade's hospital in Azad, responsible for the 4th, 5th and 6th battalions of the Brigade. I was also responsible for the headquarters and areas that reached all the way to Sul.

Our makeshift hospital was buckling at the seams. We needed something more robust if we were going to function effectively. Quickly I found another building for a new hospital; the only cement building in the village – the primary school. The principal reasoned that the war was probably going to force them to close the school year anyway, and so the job began of converting it into a hospital. Even though it was bombed regularly by the Susei garrison, I was delighted with my piece of new real estate. There were five large rooms, and one smaller room. Importantly it was clean, the floors were cemented, and the rooms had big windows and doors. The school children (mainly boys) moved the desks, blackboards, books and files to a new (and considerably less comfortable) location for the school in a matter of only hours. With the money I'd received from the commander I ordered the local tailor to make up twelve mattresses, and employed a further twelve villagers in various capacities.

Although the war had not yet started sending us casualties, primarily because the fighting in the Azad area had barely started at that point, I was still seeing over two hundred patients a day. One that particularly sticks out in my mind is that of a twenty-year-old man with lung tuberculosis combined with massive urinary bleeding. Like so many others I had seen, he was only skin and bone. In fact he was so weak that he needed to be carried in by three other men. I had never seen a patient with this ailment in such shocking condition before. I explained to his mother that the man needed to be isolated from other patients, but she flatly refused, seeing this as an insult.

"He is my only son. Better that he die than you isolate him," she told me curtly.

What a dreadful state of affairs this was. The hospital had no isolation wards to put the patient in, in fact there were no wards to speak of whatsoever. I hoped the mother might know somewhere he could be isolated, but clearly that was not to be. With some trepidation I asked the mother if she or any other members of the family were showing any symptoms of the disease. She told me they weren't, but I should have known better. Within four months both the mother and the young daughter came to me needing treatment for the same condition. I really didn't believe I could save her son; his condition was the worst I had ever seen. The poor man weighed only thirty-five kilos. I instructed the mother to give him lots of fresh air, plenty of sleep, as much meat as they could get their hands on, and under no circumstances was he to do any kind of work. Aside from that, all I could do was ask that he be brought to me on a daily basis for an injection.

For the next two months the young man was brought to me, wrapped in a blanket, by mule, on a daily basis. After only two weeks the massive urinary bleeding had stopped, but he was still too weak to stand on his own two feet. Three months later, that changed. From looming under the giant shadowy wings of the angel of death, and under the most primitively adverse conditions I'd ever want to contemplate, with love, determination and care, this young man was

65

literally brought back from the dead. Such was the nature of my work in Azad. I never knew what unfathomable challenge lay ahead, and I had long since given up trying to second guess what the fates had in store for me. For example, one day Diman came to me with a letter from the commander who had been so kind. It read as follows:

Dear Diman,
As soon as this letter reaches you, you and brother doctor must come immediately to Surdash. I have sent three Pesh Merga to accompany you.
Cordially,
Commander of Ruzgari Brigade
P.S. Hire a mule for brother doctor.

Diman suggested whatever I was required for must be of the utmost importance by the tone of the note, but at the same time he was concerned that I was up to the trip.

"If it's that important, of course I'll go," I told him firmly. "But can you be sure this letter is really from the commander?"

"Oh yes," Diman answered confidently. "It's his handwriting, and his signature is most distinctive. Besides, he has sent three of his personal Pesh Merga."

Well, who was I to argue with that?

While Diman organized some mules, I wrote instructions for my absence. Adil would be in charge of the hospital, aided by Bahnaz. I packed a bag of medicine, such as was available, with no idea of what to expect at the front. Under a moonless, freezing night we headed off down a narrow, muddy, rocky, slippery path that we could barely even see. Two Pesh Merga took the point, while one kept up the rear. I'd never attempted such a trek on a moonless night before. Even the well-trained mules were having difficulty finding a safe place to put their feet. I lost count of how many times I fell, fortunately never causing any serious damage.

"How do you keep your footing so well?" I asked Diman.

He smiled back at me. "In time you will be able to walk as well as this, brother doctor."

I didn't share his confidence, but the compliment was flattering.

The road rose higher and became colder as we neared the Daban Mountain. My extremities were so icy I couldn't feel them. Even though past experience had taught me it was colder on a mule's back, I decided this was my best course of action regardless. How the wounded managed to ride mules for hours, and sometimes days, was a fact that never ceased to amaze me. These were truly a stoic and determined people. As I sat astride the mule, I considered the three Pesh Merga who had been sent to escort us. They had trudged sixteen hours to bring me this message from the commander, and after less than an hour they had turned around to make the return journey with us. I don't know any 'regular' person who could stay awake that long, even under ideal conditions – and these were far from those! I wondered quietly to myself if the Kurdish people, and particularly the Pesh Merga, were perhaps part mountain goat!

Ever higher, ever colder, eventually I dismounted my steed and returned to foot trudging. At the summit it was incredibly windy, the only sign of life being a few lights in the village of Sadalha below. This was the headquarters of the 4th battalion of the Ruzgari brigade led by my friend Kurdo. The road was relatively bright, which only part way compensated for the fact that it was replete with numerous almost vertical curves. On reaching the summit I felt I had earned the right to ask the Pesh Merga why we were making this journey to Surdash. They told me they didn't know, but that the dresser of Sadalha had already been dispatched to the region. It was mystifying.

In Sadalha we took a brief break – brief enough for me to light a cigarette and head off again before it was even finished! I did not know where these people found their stamina. This time we were on a road that led between parallel chains of the Pira Magron and Daban mountains. Fortunately the government had not yet managed to establish a military outpost at this end of the trail. In some parts the road was hilly, but otherwise it was surprisingly, and very welcomingly, flat. It was, naturally, wet and muddy. But flat, wet and muddy was considered a luxury compared to some of the terrain I'd been forced to cover.

It was six in the morning when we finally arrived at Surdash. The early hour did nothing to dissuade me from heading straight for the commander's headquarters, and neither did the heavily-armed guards outside. They said something in the Badinan dialect that I didn't understand, but Diman replied advising them that the commander was urgently awaiting our arrival. After our shoes (but not weapons) were removed, we were cordially invited inside. The commander of the 3rd battalion, Anwar, was sitting on the floor with a cup of tea in front of him. His dark-set eyes and somber expression told me immediately that he hadn't slept all night. Slowly he looked up at us and lit a cigarette before speaking in raspy Arabic.

"The army has made an unexpected move from Kirkuk. There has been heavy fighting with the 3rd battalion. Many of our people have been killed; many more wounded, among those the battalion's commander. All through the night I've been receiving telegrams asking for medicines."

"What sort of medicines were they asking for?" I wanted to know.

He handed me a piece of paper with the Kurdish word for pethidine.

"What is this?" he asked me.

"A strong pain killer. A very strong pain killer." I paused. "But we don't have any."

"The situation is grave," the commander said simply. "There are not enough qualified dressers, and the nearest doctor can't be reached. He's probably visiting relatives," he added disapprovingly. "I had no other choice but to send for you. I know you are busy in Azad, but you are needed urgently in Kara Getan. As soon as the commander's health permits, you must bring him back here. My car will take you part of the way. I've assigned twelve Pesh Merga to take you on the rest of the journey by foot."

Diman and I were fed a hurried breakfast, and unceremoniously crammed into a land-rover with the twelve Pesh Merga, among them Diman's brothers. It didn't take long for the orchestra of death to begin ringing around us. A continuous artillery duel was being fought between the Susei garrison and the Pesh Merga. The guerillas were thousands of meters high, so the army's bombardments were little more than a futile show of strength, but they were relentless nonetheless. Although we came within meters of the garrison we were hidden behind some hills, and in any event no one seemed to take any notice of our presence. It was the first time I had been this close to the actual war, but there was no time and no room for fear. I did what everyone else did, simply what needed to be done.

To get into the village of Kara Getan we could have opted for the short route, but it might have been very short indeed, as it would take us directly into the path of the garrison. Instead we chose the 'scenic' route, an additional six-hour march in two-man formation through muddy grain fields. The only advantage of the mud was that it prevented tanks or armed cars from following us. I held onto that thought as my rubber shoes were sucked off or stuck with each new step I took. En route I noticed men, women and children digging holes in the muddy hillside.

"What are they doing that for?" I asked Diman.

"These people have seen war before," he explained. "They know with the coming spring the aircraft will start flying again. They will not be safe in their homes. They will live here until the harvest – if the government doesn't burn it first."

I gazed upon these brave and determined people with bewildered sadness as we continued our dreadful trek to comfort and aid the wounded. A few of the villagers turned to shout their encouragement,

"The Kurds will be free!"

I hoped that was a prophecy.

CHAPTER SEVEN

It was one o'clock on a gloomy afternoon when we stealthily entered the village. We took great pains to ensure the nearby garrison didn't spot us, not only for our own safety, but certain in the knowledge that should we be spotted the defenseless village would be shelled mercilessly. An old man, almost a caricature of the long struggle, invited us into his humble home. Despite our protests that we didn't have the time, he insisted.

"We'd best accept his invitation," Diman whispered to me. "These people are the kindest and bravest in all Kurdistan. It would be an insult to refuse his hospitality."

Clearly I was not to be permitted to break with tradition, so against my better judgment I entered the old man's home. Glancing around, I quickly noticed three women, the youngest maybe fourteen years old, all dressed in black. Gradually I came to realize that all the women in the area wore only black. There were no young men, they were all either dead or Pesh Merga.

We were treated to the familiar bread, yogurt, and tea before being permitted to continue on our way with fresh mules. I opted to ride this time. It was still cold, but the wind had dropped and the sun had come out – what luxury! I remained astride my trusty steed until Diman turned to me.

"Brother doctor, I think you should dismount while we cross the road. We are close to the garrison and you will be clearly spotted on the mule."

My feet were so sore I almost didn't care any more.

"Let them try," I hissed. "I'm staying on the mule." Perhaps some of the creature's stubborn nature was rubbing off on me? I neither knew nor cared, and amazingly I managed to remain astride without incident. It wasn't until we reached the battalion that I fully realized how foolish and selfish that decision had been.

The 3rd battalion's headquarters in a large yard was full of despondent looking Pesh Merga. What was it that compelled mankind to turn against brother so bitterly? Why are we constantly so driven to cause pain and suffering to the fellow inhabitants of our planet? Was there ever a time when the suffering would end? I couldn't help but let these melancholy thoughts momentarily fill my head, before chastising myself, remembering there was an urgent task at hand.

Removing our shoes we entered the commander's room. He was lying in bed, being attended to by two dressers, and surrounded by many people. As soon as he spotted me he tried to stand. Quickly I rushed to his side to prevent the futile and potentially damaging movement. Although we were strangers, we kissed in greeting, as was customary, before I was able to examine him. He looked pale, and profoundly sad, but otherwise he didn't seem to be in too bad a shape.

"How do you feel?" I asked.

"Very well," he insisted. "But these two," he pointed to the dressers, "have refused to let me eat or drink since I was wounded yesterday. They keep saying I have to wait until brother doctor arrives. And I have to tell you – I'm hungry!"

I turned to the dressers. "Is there an abdominal wound?"

"We're not certain, brother doctor. But we knew you were coming and wanted to be cautious."

I frowned. "Do you have a stethoscope?"

"What for?" a dresser asked me. "We wouldn't know what to do with it."

It was an honest answer. I took a few instruments out of my medical bag and began my examination. The commander had a bullet hole in his upper right abdomen, just below the ribs. It wasn't deep, and every other indication led me to believe the condition was quite minor in the scheme of things.

"You can eat and drink as much as you want," I told him cheerfully.

"I'm delighted to hear it, brother doctor," he smiled.

"Diman, send a telegram to the commander of the Brigade," I instructed. "Tell him the commander of the 3rd battalion is in good shape and we'll be leaving for Surdash tomorrow."

"Right away, brother doctor," my assistant replied enthusiastically.

For the time being the best prescription was bed rest, while I used the remaining time to instruct the dressers in the use of a stethoscope. It hadn't been the first time I had seen wounded denied food and drink by dressers who thought they were being prudent with the patient's health. I needed to explain that often this action could be causing more harm than good.

∞∞

My time on the front lines did bare some fruit. I managed to pick up some steel beds for the hospital, a few new dressers, and a dentist. After organizing the medical corps of the Brigade, not only did my staff complement swell, but I also received a boost to my medical and instruments supplies due to the benevolent assistance of a fellow doctor. I assigned three dressers to each battalion and two dressers to run the dispensary in Sargelow, an important town that later became the headquarters of the Brigade. A fellow doctor accepted the offer to open a hospital in Askar, where the 1st, 2nd and 5th battalions could be more adequately serviced. In my main hospital I had Adil, Diman, Bahnaz, Sherko, Serwan, Admad, Omar, Hamid, and Serwan who respectively had roles as my assistant, dressers, a pharmacist, a dentist, a lab technician, and a clerk. It was beginning to feel as though we were running a real hospital.

Everything needed to be documented, and a filing system established. At times this did burden us under a sea of paperwork, which I felt was superfluous to the revolution, but if something were to happen to me it was of paramount importance that anyone stepping into my shoes would understand the nuances of this vital machine. With new steel beds we were also finally able to set up wards, complete with not only mattresses I'd had the local tailor make, but also sheets, pillows and even blankets donated to us by the commander. The weather was getting a little warmer, which was both a blessing and a curse. The increase in the barometer meant there was less chance of freezing to death, but it also meant the bomber planes were going to start flying again. Fearing a bombardment, villagers often headed into the mountains during the day. Some would head back after sunset to spend the night in their warm homes, while others decided it was safer to remain out of sight. But to every cloud there is a silver lining. One of the permanently deserted homes became a functional dormitory for hospital personnel.

The home was old and decrepit, but at least it had a roof. It too had once been used as a stable, although when we moved in it was more like the local Hilton for indigenous reptiles. Snakes, why did it have to be snakes? I lost count of how many I saw surreptitiously slithering in and out of the nooks and crannies of deserted buildings in Azad. The important thing, however, was that this two-storey building was close to the hospital. On colder nights medical personnel would sleep in the two rooms upstairs, but as soon as the mercury rose they felt happier sleeping outside in the yard. For myself, I rented a room in a building next door, the walls of which were covered with old newspaper. Perhaps ironically this gave me a chance to catch up on some news. Although they were out of date they were my only contact with the outside world apart from a little radio I'd managed to obtain.

The outside yard of the old building was surrounded by a 1.5 meter high wall, which gave us the illusion of security and privacy. It was here we set up our kitchen with enough dishes, pots and pans to cater for thirty people. The meals were, almost needless to say, very humble. Breakfast usually consisted of bread and tea. Lunch and dinner were feasts of grain (usually rice) with a vegetable stew – and more bread and tea. Once a week we were sometimes able to secure some meat, such as turkey or mutton. Occasionally we had a rare treat of beef or goat.

We hadn't long moved into this palatial edifice when we received our first ward case. A twelve-year-old girl had been bitten by a snake in the village of Omar Kom, between Surdash and Sadalah. The venom had already been in her system for a day when she reached me, causing massive internal bleeding. Her legs were so swollen they looked like two puffed up balloons, and her abdomen was rigid. I sighed quietly with a heavy heart. There was no way this little life could be saved, the poison was already too far advanced in her system. It would have taken many pints of valuable blood to simply delay the inevitable. Sadly I told her father what my prognosis was, wishing there was some way I could perform a miracle. Of course this was not to be and early the following morning I was called to the hospital to witness the poor child's death. Even though it was hopeless I started mouth-to-mouth resuscitation to show the dressers who had gathered how it should be done. Her father stood quietly by, while her young heartsick brother couldn't contain his grief.

The girl was buried in a cemetery behind the hospital. Many of the local villagers, who were complete strangers to this family, turned up with shovels asking to help. No one was crying any longer, not even her small brother. They had all seen so much death it was as though they had no tears left to cry, yet they would never turn their back when it came to helping a fellow soul – even a complete stranger. I wondered for a time why the girl wasn't taken to her home town for burial. When I quietly asked one of my colleagues about this the answer seemed painfully obvious. These people had long ago learned that in death, as in life, they had to be practical. Death was a part of life, and life goes on.

The second ward patient I treated brought no respite from the dark cloud of dismal death. He was a young man, around twenty-six years old, who was so painfully thin, anemic, and weak that he could hardly stand or talk. His liver and spleen were enlarged, and for a few weeks he'd been suffering from fever, malaise, nose bleeds, and jaundice. More recently his stomach had become enlarged, and he was experiencing joint pain and a loss of appetite. Serwan said he could run tests on the red and white blood cell count, along with a general urine examination. Within an hour he had the results back, written in English (which I think he felt very proud of). I studied Serwan's findings before turning slowly towards the man with sympathetic eyes.

"Have you heard of leukemia?" I asked softly.

He looked at me with sad, dark, tired eyes. "Isn't that cancer of the blood?"

I nodded and took his hand. All I was able to do was draw up an intensive care plan. Further tests revealed he was also suffering from malaria. We gave him penicillin, high doses of cortisone and tonics. In addition I prescribed digoxin for his swollen legs. Over the following three weeks I was able to improve his general condition to a level where he was strong enough to return to his home, a two-day ride from the village of Azad. A month later word reached me that he died a week after he'd returned to his family.

With increasing numbers of serious cases came increasing problems. It was customary in Iraq for a family to stay with a sick person in order to carry out the manual chores required to care for the ailing. The obvious advantage of this was that it removed pressure from the minimal staff I had, but on the other hand family members took up room by sleeping on the floor by their relatives, and they required feeding, which used valuable resources. Eventually I had to forbid this practice, instead teaching my dressers the finer points of ward sanitation and patient care. It took some time for them to accept this concept, but eventually they could see the wisdom in my suggestion and conducted themselves like thorough professionals.

I'd often wondered silently what would happen if my hospital was bombed when the waiting room was full to overflowing with people. On the 24th of April, 1974, that picture was painted all too gruesomely for me…

At 9:45am, two Sukhoi 7 fighter bombers attacked the town of Qualat Dizah with five hundred and fifty pound bombs. Their targets were the crowded center of town, a makeshift university building, a hospital, and a school. There were over three hundred casualties: one hundred and thirty-four killed, and two hundred wounded – mainly women, children, and university students. The grisly statistics that filtered through to me clinically announced that among the dead and wounded were a number of hospital patients and personnel. Over one hundred homes were damaged or destroyed. On top of that the bombers decimated public buildings including the Tobacco Monopoly Office, the hospital, the municipality center, the Mayor's home, the town's public bath, the Qualat Dizah Hotel, the school, the power station, and parts of the makeshift university. Forty-seven shops, tea rooms, and restaurants were also obliterated, burying both the owners and their patrons under rubble. The following day seven hundred students and thirty professors abandoned their plans for further studies, most of them choosing to join the Pesh Merga.

It was this tragedy that prompted me to change my hospital's schedule. I decided that less serious cases would only be seen at night, announcing I would open for business at 6pm daily, and not close my doors again until two hundred patients had been cared for. An unfortunate side-effect of this schedule was that people traveling from other villages had to spend much of the night traveling home again, for only under the cover of darkness was it safe to move around any longer.

Even with our increased facilities we were still woefully short of equipment that would be considered commonplace in normal hospitals. Due to this fact when the commander of the important and famous Ruzgari Brigade was brought to me with a massive swelling in his right knee, I was unable to X-ray him. Despite my suggestion that he head to Galala, he refused. Only when the 4th medical section was opened in Pen Jewin did he agree to travel for more advanced treatment. As a result he was kept away from playing an active role in the battle that ensued. It was also around this time that we received our first wounded Pesh Merga. Two men, both around thirty-five years of age, were brought to us from the 5th battalion. One had an upper arm fracture and a shrapnel wound high in his chest. This was the fifth time he'd been injured in battle. Usually, in a case such as this, an operation would be carried out and the bone fixed. However, due to our shortage of instruments we had no other choice other than to try and fix his arm with plaster cast.

I could feel my nose wrinkle as an offensive odor wafted through my olfactory senses, indicating the wound was infected. Without any local anesthetic I cut it, cleaned it, and sewed some adaption stitches. From there I put a very stable plaster cast around it. On examining his shrapnel wound I decided it posed too much of a risk to try and remove it, as without X-ray equipment it was impossible to determine exactly where it was. Fortunately I could tell his lung had not been damaged. I treated him as well as I was able with the facilities at my disposal, and turned my attention to his comrade.

The other Pesh Merga had a tiny hole below the navel. He looked pale and disorientated, and told me he'd had no stool for the past four days. His blood pressure and pulse were normal, with a temperature reading of 38oC. All oral intake, be it food, water, or medicines, had to be stopped. The patient could only be kept alive with infusions of glucose water, and we only had 500ml of that in stock. In addition there was no infusion system ready, so I started his treatment by giving him glucose water with a 10ml syringe. If I could keep him from taking anything orally for a day there was a chance I could reach a final diagnosis. Meanwhile I sent Hama, one of my staff, to the dispensary at Jawarta, telling him to bring back as many infusions as he could carry.

The next morning there was no real improvement in the Pesh Merga's condition, and no sign of Hama. My patient looked dry, pale and toxic. He insisted he was feeling well, and wanted something to eat and drink. In 2005 we live in times of wondrous technology, but in 1974 there was no means by which I could contact Hama. Oh for a cell phone to call and ask where he was, and how long he would be. But back in 1974 in Kurdistan no such technology was available. I had no way of knowing when, or if, Hama would be back. By the afternoon I decided to let the Pesh Merga have some tea, which I fed him with a spoon. Overnight I saw a further two hundred patients. Only after I'd completed my surgery was I able to return to the Pesh Merga to check on his condition. He had had plenty of tea, but he still looked toxic and his temperature still read 38oC. I just didn't have the proper instruments to attempt surgery, to do so would have almost certainly meant death for the patient. I could only watch and wait and pray and care for the man the best I was able.

The following morning Hama reappeared with eight pints of glucose water 5% and normal saline. Apparently at Jawarta they were also out of infusions, so he'd been sent to Moutat, a further twelve hours away. My dedicated team member did not stop traveling until he'd secured all that was on offer and returned back to me, utterly exhausted. Eight pints wasn't much, but the doctor in Moutat was a friend of mine, and had given Hama all he had available. I began the infusions immediately, but it was plain to see this stock was not going to be sufficient. The abdominal injury was localized with an abscess forming in the lower abdominal area. It took three days until we were able to send him to the 4th section hospital, which had just opened. The transportation itself presented us with yet a new challenge. By now there were several injured Pesh Merga in my care who could be better treated in the 4th section hospital, but to get them there safely they needed to travel horizontally. It's incredible how creative one can become when faced with impossible challenges.

Necessity truly is the mother of invention. To transport the wounded we fixed a coffin firmly onto one mule's back, and put the injured man inside. Another mule was fixed with a ladder, and a reasonably comfortable mattress tied astride it. Wherever there was a challenge, there was also a solution, even if it did take Ahmed three and a half days to eventually get all the injured men across to Pen Jewin. The chief surgeon there operated immediately, saving all but the man with the stomach injury. He died in hospital. With no close relatives to speak of his personal belongings were sent back to us. I studied these meager symbols of a man's entire life: a wristwatch, a wallet with twelve pounds, and his weapon, all of which we returned to his battalion. Later I was to learn the circumstances under which these brave men had been wounded...

In early April the Brigade received information that the army was moving a large force from Kirkuk to Sul, intending to reinforce its troops in the Susei garrison and establishing outposts in the areas in between. A Special Pesh Merga unit, one hundred men strong, led by Kurdo, had a plan to halt their advance near Chemen, twelve kilometers from Kirkuk. The men were ordered to rendezvous at Tilyan, around a day's walk from Chemen. It was raining heavily – again. After a day's walk through muddy, hilly countryside they still had a long and arduous march ahead, therefore when they approached Chemen the battle had already begun. Fifty Pesh Merga had dug in positions on both sides of the highway. The rain was unrelenting, yet nothing could blockade the brave, skilled and determined Pesh Merga Special Forces from pushing into battle. By the time the unit with my patients reached the fray around three hundred Pesh Merga were involved, armed mainly with burno rifles, a few automatic weapons, and two hundred and twenty bullets. They also had two RBGs and one artillery piece.

It was a code of honor with the Pesh Merga that none would leave the fighting before sunset, even if their ammunition supply had been exhausted. They had no food, and no medical supplies. By contrast, the army had a Brigade of four thousand well-equipped soldiers with five hundred Kurdish mercenaries and Special Forces in front of their convoy. They were also outfitted with several armed cars, tanks and artillery units – all the very latest Russian apparatus. If it sounds a little imbalanced, a little like the Pesh Merga were up against impossible odds, then add into the mix that the army was also flying bomber planes, and to psych up their soldiers the army claimed the Pesh Merga were two thousand strong, well-equipped with modern weapons, and that they were barricaded into well-dug positions. This piece of intell came to me from an army officer who later deserted to join the Movement.

The battle raged throughout the day, despite the non-stop deluge from heaven. Only after the sunset did the main Pesh Merga force withdraw to a deserted village to spend the night on the cold floor of a Mosque, soaked through and with no food. Their Special Forces meanwhile kept guard on the highway, as the army continued shelling the surrounding villages throughout the night. It is hard, if not impossible, to imagine what it was like trying to get some sleep on a cold stone floor, utterly exhausted, soaked to the bone, hungry for food that would not be forthcoming, and hearing shells exploding all around you, before returning at sunrise to join the Pesh Merga brethren.

Come morning both the rain and the shells were still falling. Against overwhelming odds the Pesh Merga held their ground, even though by sunset the following evening they were running out of ammunition, and they'd been without food for two days. A strategic decision was made to withdraw to Jamjamal where the 4th battalion was waiting for the advancing army. The battle could be continued there.

By the third day of battle it was reported that only four Pesh Merga had been killed, as opposed to fifty-three from the army. Devoid of food or sleep the Special Forces marched all day to reach

Jamjamal. The fighting continued for a further two days, although casualties on both sides were surprisingly moderate. As the army advanced onto the town of Taslogah, around twenty-five kilometers from Sul, the Pesh Merga desperately needed rest and sustenance. The 2nd, 3rd and 4th battalions of Pesh Merga rostered their units in turn to tackle the government's forces. By the thirteenth day the army retreated to the village of Derbanbazyan, between Taslogah and Jamjamal. In this battle my friend Kurdo was severely injured, his left arm receiving major nerve damage, yet his fighting spirit was undaunted. Such is the spirit of a man fighting to defend his home, his land, and all that he believes in more than life itself.

CHAPTER EIGHT

In among all this brutality and horror I decided to create something that was both beautiful and practical. Partly this was for my sanity, but equally it would provide an enormous benefit for the patients in my care. I wanted to build a garden – a big, bold, beautiful vegetable garden. But how?

I took Diman aside one night and began to explore the possibilities.

"Do you think it would be possible for me to rent a piece of land from one of the villagers?" I asked him tentatively.

"Possibly," he mused. "The villagers don't cultivate their land during war. Why? What do you have in mind?"

I explained my plan, suggesting I could hire one of the villagers to help me take care of it.

"It sounds like a wonderful idea," Diman gushed. "I'll look into it right away."

Within a day he'd found a suitable piece of soil for me; a plot owned by a young man whose father had just died.

"I would be willing to rent you the land for a year," the young man said simply.

"How much do you want for it?"

"As it's for the hospital, I will charge you just ten pounds for the year."

"It's a deal," I smiled.

The property was perfect: two thousand square meters situated on the safer side of the village and surrounded by a wall of high trees. There was a gate into the property and a large stream of fresh water around the entire area. The soil itself was in good condition, as it had been planted the year before and there were very few worms to worry about. Although in truth, worms were the least of our concern. Bahanz had enough DDT to kill off every worm in Azad! Quickly work began on my dream of a little piece of paradise in the middle of the jaws of hell. I hired Karim, a local villager, as he had two cows with which he could prepare the land for planting. While his cows ploughed, Bahnaz set to work spraying the area with a thick layer of DDT. Within what seemed merely the blink of an eye we were seeding tomatoes, okra, green beans, peppers, onions, eggplants, watermelon, honey melon, and countless other vegetables. My joy was soon overshadowed by shame, however, when I shot a black snake that silently slithered through my sanctuary.

Karim came running as soon as he heard my pistol discharge. In my mind, having seen the ugly and fatal effects of snakebites, the only good snake was a dead snake. Karim looked upon the lifeless corpse of the indigenous reptile with wiser eyes. Seeing my bullet lodged squarely in the center of its skull, Karim told me accusingly that although these snakes were deadly, they never attacked humans. Like other creatures in this land, they were hungry. Our ploughing had stirred up the worms, a healthy meal for a starving snake. All the poor creature was doing was looking for a meal. Furthermore, he would have helped rid our land of any worms that the DDT didn't take care of. I was humbled and ashamed at how little I understood of the ways of these people.

Daily I would wander into my little paradise, careful never to harm another living thing, tingling with anticipation of the new life this venture would bring forth. The tiny little tomato plants that began to sprout looked so helpless in their new home I only hoped Karim's expert care would ensure their survival. Even though I had high expectations for this ambitious venture, I was both astonished and delighted when a few weeks later the whole area was a thriving mass of green, healthy plants. Day by day my magic garden grew stronger and healthier, to the point where a sea of green was visible from quite a distance away. It was therapeutic for everyone, becoming an idyllic location to escape from the horrors for just a little while, soaking in the sensually exquisite aromas of fresh and flourishing new life.

When the harvest came it was with abundance. We were rewarded for our labors over a period of months with hundreds of kilos of produce. Every item was a prized and rare delicacy as nothing so extravagant was brought in from the cities. There were fresh vegetables for patients and staff alike. For the undernourished wounded it was a banquet fit for a king.

∞∞

Months into the war it was still only warming up on many fronts, although there were already many casualties on both sides. However, this did nothing to dampen the spirit of hope among my Kurdish brethren. We all knew we were in this for the long haul.

The government's wounded were taken to military hospitals in the north until they could hold no more. As the war progressed, and hospitals could no longer cope, any facility that could be seized was used as a hospital (and where the government was concerned they could seize anything they wanted). Of course Baghdad tried to disguise their number of casualties. Across time it has been known that the first casualty of war is the truth. Identification numbers were taken from soldiers by the government; if they were killed in battle it would hence be impossible for Kurds to broadcast their names over the radio. When families inquired about a missing son they were either told that the authorities didn't know what had become of him, or alternatively they were told that Kurds had killed him while captive. Both stories were lies. The government well knew what happened to their soldiers, and no Kurd I had dealings with ever killed a captive soldier.

In truth many of the government's military preferred life as a Prisoner Of War, because for them the war was over. It was a war most of them didn't believe in to start with, but due to the fascist controlled government in Baghdad they had no choice but to fight – to kill, or be killed. Hundreds of dead and wounded government soldiers were just left on the battlefields. The Kurdish leadership had given a standing order to the Pesh Merga to bury any such poor souls they came across. As none of the fallen were permitted identification cards they were all buried according to the Islamic faith, even though many of them were Christians. The government did concede to return fallen officers to their families, but public funerals were forbidden. Many brave Iraqis ignored this demand by Baghdad, risking their own lives to give an appropriate farewell to those they loved, those who had been lost in a futile and unjust battle.

Inevitably the death toll rose, and with it the popularity of my hospital increased. An ironic outcome of this situation was the ever-growing number of women who felt they could ask for medical aid. I remember one particular case of a man bursting into my hospital weeping, "Brother doctor, please come quickly. My wife, she is very sick and needs your help."

"What is she suffering from?" I asked.

"It is her pregnancy? She is so pale and weak."

"Is she bleeding?" I asked, thinking this was a reasonable question. As I watched the man I could swear he started to blush.

"I think so," he replied sheepishly.

"What month is she in?"

"I don't know. Maybe the fourth or fifth."

"You must bring her to the hospital immediately," I told him sternly.

"Oh, brother doctor," the man gasped. "Her mother would not let her come here – and her brothers. You know how people here think. They would never let her come to the hospital for such a thing."

"You and your wife need to make this decision," I replied firmly. "All women here are considered our own mothers and sisters. If you need help to get her here I can send a Pesh Merga to assist."

The man looked horrified, but I convinced him to consider the option. Diman returned to the man's home with him to take the woman's blood pressure and assess the situation. Watching them leave I couldn't help but wonder about a people whose honor meant more to them than the life of a female loved one. To have a male examine a female, even a male doctor, was considered shameful, yet they were prepared to permit such assistance if it could be kept completely clandestine. This villager had six children to care for, and he was prepared to risk all of them, for they would surely suffer without their mother's care, rather than risk dishonor.

I busied myself with my other patients, not noticing how much time had passed when Diman came running back out of breath.

"Brother doctor! The woman is very sick. I could not measure her blood pressure but her mother tells me she's been bleeding for three days."

For a moment I didn't realize the husband was standing behind Diman, almost in tears.

"Please, brother doctor," the man begged. "Please save my wife for the sake of our other children. I don't care what people say."

Apparently Diman had talked sense to the man. I immediately dispatched four of our people and a stretcher to fetch the woman. I didn't exactly have anything that would pass as a gynecological table so I set about creating a makeshift piece of apparatus that would do the job; a table with two 60cm long pieces of thick wood tied to the sides. Linen cloth was nailed to the boards enabling us to keep her legs separated by tying them to the planks of wood, but I did not have all the necessary instruments to clear out a bleeding uterus and no infusions or anesthesia.

The instruments we had were boiled in preparation for the woman's arrival. She was so weak that fortunately there was no need for any narcosis. She was also deeply in shock, but my first priority had to be to stop the bleeding. I kept Diman and Adil in the surgery, such as it was, and instructed everyone else to leave, closing the door behind them. The situation was fraught with danger, not least of which due to the fact it was mid afternoon – a prime time for aerial bombers.

"Tell her not to be afraid," I told Diman. "Tell her we consider her our sister."

Diman repeated my words in her native tongue but I don't think they registered. She just lay there, utterly motionless.

Sterilization of both ourselves and the operating area consisted of washing in soap, water and antiseptic. Surgical gloves were a luxury we did not possess. The patient was in complete abortion, bleeding heavily, and her cervix was fully dilated. It took me five minutes or so to clear out more than half a pint of coagulated blood, placenta, and pieces of her unborn fetus. An offensive odor told me infection has already set in. I had no sooner cleaned out the uterus when fresh bubbling blood started pouring out; a sign that usually means the uterus is empty.

Diman was instructed to massage the uterus externally from the abdomen. That halted the bleeding, allowing us to give her an injection and rest for a while. An hour later there was still no sign of bleeding, but before I called in her family I was careful to wash, dispose of, or hide any bloody evidence that an abortion had taken place.

A week later I visited the woman in her home. Happily she'd made a full recovery, but I told her she wasn't to have any more babies while the war continued.

"But my husband might marry another woman," she laughed.

Apparently birth control pills were unheard of in this area, and even if they had been heard of they would have been forbidden. Nonetheless, when I managed to get my hands on some I quickly had fifty women taking them. That first gynecological case opened the way for many women to at least feel they could more freely ask for my assistance, and over time I even developed a bona fide gynecological examination room with a delivery section.

On one of the rare occasions it was sunny, Adil and I were busy working on case sheets when Darwish came bursting in with blood all over his face and his fingers in his ears.

"Come out fast! Two planes…"

He hadn't finished his sentence when massive explosions shook the building, blowing the windows clean out. We raced outside to see a huge cloud of smoke on the other side of the village where most of the homes were located.

"There will be injured," Adil said sadly.

"We'd best go and see," I agreed.

The in-house patients were all moved to as safe a location as we could find on a moment's notice, and we ran to where the village had been bombed. The sight that met my eyes was sickening. At first it didn't all sink in. I felt tears welling as I scanned the panorama to see nothing but a twisted mass of upturned earth, wood and stones. The two bombers had hit their mark with deadly precision. Every home in the area had been completely destroyed. I prayed quickly and quietly that the villagers had not been inside when this disaster struck. Gazing over the rubble it was as though time stood still. A smoky haze filled the landscape. It could have been the terrain as it was before the birth of life on earth – or long after it had all been destroyed.

Gradually one dazed face after another began to emerge from the destruction. The people had happily managed to reach safety before the bombs struck, and now they were all focused on just one thing – to get back to their livestock who'd been in the yards when the devastation hit.

"Please don't," I urged. "There could be unexploded bombs."

Sadly heeding our advice the villagers waited until it was considered safe before they began digging for their animals. Eight cows and a mule were discovered mangled in the wreckage. The most prudent advice I was able to give was to burn the carcasses to prevent the spread of disease. It was meager comfort indeed. Preventing disease meant little when their very livelihood had been lost.

Trekking back to the hospital my steps were leaden. My whole being was weighed with the knowledge that we could no longer remain where we were. As if to confirm my grim prophecy, en route back I happened across a tiny kitten. The dear little defenseless soul had blood coming from its ears. Many of the children of Qualat Dizah had suffered the same fate. The force of these bombs sent shock waves so severe they could easily cause a cerebral hemorrhage to small children and animals even if they weren't actually struck by the explosion.

The kitten was dead.

The children of Qualat Dizah were dead.

The lifetime of my hospital on its current location was dead.

How much death can one person witness and remain sane? It's a question I cannot answer.

My patients were still hiding in the mountains, many of them in plaster casts. The whole village was deserted. Only after sunset did the scene change. As if emerging from a mirage, suddenly everywhere sprang back into life. It was bizarre bordering on surreal, but this is how it would have to be until I secured a safer location for the hospital. Patients would have to be hidden by day, and returned at night. I would have to organize a new facility with great haste.

Setting off on my search I climbed a nearby hill to determine a good location for the summer hospital only to spot twenty Pesh Merga heading towards Azad. I quickly scuttled back to the hospital, noticing they had a wounded man astride a mule. There could be little doubt of their intended destination. Sure enough we arrived at my facility almost simultaneously. I watched with little surprise as the wounded man was brought to me, thinking he looked strikingly like Hemingway.

"This is Hagi Karim," I was told.

"It's just a small leg injury," he barked. "Nothing serious.

I unwrapped the bloody turban that had been used as a bandage around his wound. Sure enough the wound wasn't too serious.

"That's what makes me mad," he scowled. "After three hours of heavy fighting we had driven them back and *then* I got hit in the leg! I've never been so angry in my entire life!"

I was to learn they had fought a gallant battle; twenty against three hundred. Undoubtedly such gritty resolve came from the leader down. Hagi apparently refused to take cover no matter how fierce the fighting was. He'd stand in the open and shoot at anything within range. I could only marvel at the fact that he hadn't been killed, let alone escaped with such a minor injury.

His Pesh Merga decided they would make camp in the trees in the northern part of the village. It was cold, but relatively protected. I visited him daily, gradually growing in admiration for this extraordinary man. He was not only courageous and unafraid to speak his mind, but he was also honest with a love so deep for his people that no sacrifice was too great. As soon as he was able to walk again, Hagi enjoyed visiting me in my magic garden. Perhaps it is vanity, but I glowed with pride when he told me that I'd created a wonderful thing here – here among the horror of hell. In return for my administrations, and the excursions into the green pastures of my vegetable plantation, Hagi advised me on a secure location for the summer hospital. A Brigade commander had promised us a huge tent, which may not sound very robust but when dug one and a half meters underground it felt like a mini fortress. However, the fates had yet more challenges in store for us. Before leaving, Hagi Karim presented me with his own pistol telling me, "Brother doctor, I see you don't have a pistol. Take mine. It will protect you." I carried his pistol until the last moment of the tragic breakdown.

No sooner had we started digging when Azad fell victim to the first shelling from the Susei garrison. The sickening whining of bombs screeched their death threat over the village, but ever resilient the people of Azad were not to be dissuaded. The strongest men I'd ever met, both of mind and body, dug with every ounce of strength they had to create a safe haven for our new facility. The tent, once erected underground, was almost invisible. Only its white peak popped through the surface, and that was easily camouflaged with fresh green branches. The area was surrounded by lush, high trees, heavily laden with fruit. Food for the wounded was relatively plentiful and appetizing, certainly by comparison to what they'd received at the front. We were able to serve around a hundred grams of meat to everyone three times a week, and in between there were ample supplies of rice, vegetables and bread. My gynecological ward was needless to say a casualty of this forced relocation, and that did present some complications when a young Pesh Merga came urgently seeking my advice.

"Brother doctor, my wife has been having labor pains for three days, but the baby won't come. Please will you come and see her."

The woman was hardly more than a child, an eighteen-year-old who'd left the city for the first time during the sixth month of her pregnancy. Armed with my fetus stethoscope and blood pressure apparatus I hurried with Diman to see the patient. She only lived a half hour walk from the village in an area dense with fruit trees. The property was in fact one of the most beautiful farms I'd seen, yet the couple lived in a two-man tent with hardly enough room for a third person to enter. Having said that, somehow I managed to squeeze inside with the midwife and three other women! In short order I asked the three superfluous women to wait outside, leaving only myself, the patient, and the eighty-year-old midwife, who was happily rather skinny. Without wanting to sound disrespectful, 'midwife' was probably a generous term for this woman. Her function was primarily to sit by a pregnant woman's side and encourage her until the baby was born. She did facilitate the separation of the newborn from the placenta, but that was pretty much the beginning and end of any medical expertise.

The mother-to-be hadn't eaten in three days and was clearly exhausted. Her uterus wasn't contracting sufficiently for the baby to be born. At least the fetal stethoscope confirmed the baby was alive, and its heartbeat seemed fairly regular. I instructed the midwife to collect all the pillows she could get her hands on, and I tried to walk the patient around while her makeshift delivery room was prepared. Six pillows were placed on each side of the bed to enable the young woman to elevate and spread her legs. Happily the midwife took instructions well, following up her first task by preparing hot water and clean basins when requested. Meantime I asked the young woman to empty her bladder, which she did inside the tent. At this stage of the proceedings my main concern was keeping both mother and child alive.

The young woman took up her position on the bed with her legs apart on the pillows. I gave her a strong sedative injection and rechecked the fetal heartbeat. It was still strong. The sedative took effect quickly, calming my patient and evening her breathing, but the labor was still weak. On this occasion I had the good fortune to have stocks of surgical gloves. I scrubbed, I washed in antiseptic, and I donned the gloves as Diman boiled the necessary instruments: a pair of scissors, a needle holder, a few stitching needles, and regular sewing thread. This gave time for the outer cervix to fully dilate. The frequency of labor contractions increased, but they were still weak.

"Inject five units of piton into the infusion," I told Diman. "Let the infusion run at thirty-two drops a minute."

This was an effective uterus contracting mixture. Within fifteen minutes the uterus responded nicely, contracting strongly and frequently. Half an hour later the baby was born; a healthy-looking six-pound boy – with a massive blood blister on his head. I attempted to aspirate it, but not much had come out when one of the villagers came rushing to the scene.

"Brother doctor, wounded men have arrived at the hospital and urgently need your attention."

"Of course," I muttered under my breath. "Diman, you will have to take over here. Be sure the patient isn't bleeding."

Diman had become quite an expert midwife over his tenure with me. Even if it disturbed the locals to have a man attending a woman, and one who wasn't even a qualified doctor at that, I had every confidence in him.

When I returned to the hospital it was crowded with women and children, most of them crying, and some of them with mules by their side! They knew I didn't start administrations until 6:00pm unless the need was urgent, so generally they hid out in the surrounding hills and bushes until we opened. Today it wasn't so, and chaotic didn't come close to describing it! Inside the three wounded men I rushed back for were already in the dressing room, although I'd hardly call them men. One was sixteen years old and another merely twelve. The sixteen-year-old was lying on his stomach with blood covering his rear. The twelve-year-old was sitting on a chair with a bandage around his upper right leg. The third man was wounded in the knee, and all three of them were flanked by relatives.

"Bahnaz," I sighed. "Will you please get everyone out of here who doesn't need to be in here? Have you forgotten I left strict instructions that no one is to be allowed in here during the day?"

It did feel as though I was banging my head against a proverbial wall at times. The father of one of the boys rushed up to me and kissed my hand before following my instructions.

"We have only God and you, please try and save our boy!"

I automatically withdrew my hand, but politely kissed him on the forehead.

"You needn't worry about your boy," I told him calmly. "His injuries are not serious. He's going to be fine."

Having dispersed the relatives I began examining the wounded.

"How did this happen?" I asked Bahnaz.

"They were on their way to a neighboring village when a tank opened fire on them."

"Were they carrying weapons?"

"No."

It seemed moot to ask why then the government was firing on children – they were male, they were Kurds, and they were in the wrong place at the wrong time – there need be no more reason than that.

91

The sixteen-year-old had a huge wound on his right buttock, the whole muscle was destroyed. It was also full of dirt as he'd fallen and been dragged a hundred meters. Fortunately the major tendon hadn't been damaged, but he had lost at least two pints of blood. I instructed Bahnaz to clean the wound while I examined the other two.

The twelve-year-old had been hit in the upper thigh; happily it was just a flesh wound. The third man was a fifty-year-old farmer who'd been hit just below the knee. He'd been lucky though; there didn't appear to be any nerve damage.

By the time I'd finished treating them I was late starting my evening's surgery – and the mob was restless.

I was tired.

I was very, very tired.

I was a long way from giving up or giving in, but I really wasn't sure how much longer I could maintain a pace like this – even if the conditions were ideal – and the conditions were *far* from ideal.

CHAPTER NINE

The sun rose lazily on a beautiful June day. I pondered briefly about the master plan of the cosmos, wondering if any greater power than ourselves looked down on us from somewhere, and wept for all the bitter suffering mankind endured. My self-indulgent reflection was short lived, however. As though in answer to my philosophical question another group of wounded Pesh Merga were brought into my hospital needing attention. Apparently when the Brigade headquarters was moved from Surdash to Sargelow, a few Pesh Merga were left behind to guard the remaining supplies. The army caught wind of this and attacked without mercy, using both planes and artillery from the Susei garrison. Many good men were injured, although thankfully for the main part the wounds were superficial. One exception to this good fortune occurred to a Pesh Merga who'd been inside a building when the bombs struck. Glass splinters had polka-dotted across his entire body. A few of these were deeply embedded and infected. It took two hours just to remove them all.

The demand for the summer hospital became so colossal that food and medical supplies were once again falling to critical levels. The war had spread over the length and breadth of Kurdistan, with battles raging on several fronts. As with all wars, it was brutal. Yet although the government's army outnumbered and outgunned us they were reticent to attack on all fronts simultaneously. Rather they preferred to move their full might from one battle to the next, which actually didn't win them as much ground as they might have hoped. Publicly the Ba'athists claimed that the progressive socialist Iraqi government was fighting against the agents of imperialism and the Shah of Iran. It was quite amazing how creative the mendacious rhetoric was.

93

One of the more serious cases I received during this phase was a sixty-year-old man who'd been hiding out in a cave with his family. If I'd had the time to consider the matter, it would have been quite intriguing to imagine how a shell could have found its way inside the cave, but the simple fact of the matter was – it did. A huge piece of shrapnel, about the size of a pigeon, blasted into his chest and lodged in his rib cage, incredibly without damaging any actual ribs. Between the inlet on the right side of his chest where the object was located there was a straight black line which looked like a paved street. It was so badly burned it was possible to imagine that someone had drawn on him with charcoal. But this was no drawing; this was embedded deep into the man's flesh. There was also a large bullet hole in the region of his upper abdomen. The man was sweating, having difficulty breathing, and needless to say he was in a great deal of pain.

I gave him a sedative and prepared my instruments for surgery. As I began removing the vile item I found myself wondering how something this large had managed to enter his chest and yet not damage his ribs. It was huge, and the man told me when the shrapnel entered his body, it was so hot that for hours afterwards he still felt as though his chest was on fire. He was tough though, determined to live to see a free Kurdistan. Such determination helped him withstand the surgery well, and I was able to conduct further tests which seemed to indicate that his liver had been injured. He would need to go to the 4th medical section in Pen Jewin for the rest of his treatment, which necessitated a mule ride to Kariza from where a car could be hired to take him the rest of the way. It would be a five hour journey on a stretcher fixed to a mule's back before he could travel in the relative comfort of a car. I doubt many, if any, city dwellers could have withstood the journey.

With the man safely on his way to Kariza, I conducted my evening's surgery and fell into bed hoping I wouldn't be plagued in sleep by the horrific images that met my eyes during the day.

The following day seemed full of promise. The air was sweet; the sun was shining, and the sky pristinely clear. Adil and I were en route to the hospital with Darwish when a Sukhoi 7 fighter bomber appeared from nowhere. The plane flew low between the mountains, heading straight for us.

"Hit the ground!" Darwish cried.

Scampering for cover I saw my life and the lives of my patients flashing before my eyes. Would this be the end of it? I watched, holding my breath, as the fighter whizzed over us without dropping a bomb. I dared to look up only to see he'd made a turn and was charging straight back towards us, flying low over our heads towards the village. The following seconds unfolded in slow motion as a series of huge explosions reverberated in my ears. Ominous clouds of black smoke plumed into mushroom-shaped clouds between the two mountains ahead.

"Oh God," I almost wept, seeing they'd hit the very area that many villagers had moved to, thinking they'd be safe from attack by both the garrison and the fighter planes.

The army had become wise to the fact that the village was deserted. Never wishing to miss an opportunity to take innocent lives, they'd sent their fighter planes, their devilish demons of death, to search out cattle in the surrounding areas, knowing the local people would not be far away. True to his mission, this pilot had spotted the humble homes nestled in the hillside, and dropped his payload without qualm or mercy.

Scrambling to our feet we ran towards the area of the attack, around two kilometers away. What horrors was I to witness this time? I didn't have the luxury of epoch to consider it.

We arrived in only a few minutes to be met by a scene filled with smoke and debris. My heart stopped. I held my breath, wondering what terrible fate had befallen my brethren. Squinting through the dismal mist my worst fears were happily quashed. Quickly I discovered that most of the people had scampered to safe ground before the bombs hit their mark. But the news wasn't all good. One tiny infant had died from a hemorrhage caused by the shock wave, blood trickling out of his tiny ears. Why had God given him life only to take it away again? It didn't make sense. But remorse and reflection would have to wait. A two meter long, two ton bomb had landed in a moist pasture and not yet exploded. No one would be safe until the bomb disposal experts had dismantled it. These teams were always at the ready. I wondered what they did for a profession before the war, and what they might do afterwards. Would there ever be an 'afterwards'? So many questions, so few answers.

As always, with these people, nothing would go to waste. The gunpowder the bomb disposal experts extracted would be packaged and sold to fishermen who had no other means left to secure a haul of fresh fish. For every cloud there truly seemed to be a silver lining somewhere – if only a person knew where to look for it.

∞∞

As the year ticked on the weather became ever warmer. However, the tender glow of the life-giving sun brought with it no respite for the people of Azad. With clear skies the air raids would become more frequent – and more accurate. Summer homes needed to be constructed to provide shelter for these brave people, but the only materials to hand were tree branches, and living at one with nature was accompanied by its own dangers. This was the season for snakes, scorpions, malaria carrying mosquitoes, and disease carrying rats. With no anti-venom for the snakes, and no blood transfusions possible, to be bitten by a snake was certain death. For every step we took forward it felt as though we were forced to take three steps back. At every angle there was a new challenge, a new danger, a new dilemma that required urgent attention.

It was becoming clear that unless we were fully mobile we wouldn't be safe anywhere. Government agents managed to slither into the most unexpected places to glean information and filter it back to headquarters in Baghdad. But how could I make my hospital mobile? I would have to discuss the matter with Diman as soon as he returned from Pen Jewin.

My trusty assistant had been in Pen Jewin at the 4th medical section with a patient of mine, a squadron commander with an abdominal injury. The fifty-year-old patient had arrived at my hospital deathly pale, and he appeared uncharacteristically frightened. After a brief examination it was clear he had an internal injury to the bowel, and was therefore going to need to make the trek to the 4th medical section. I sent Diman with him, along with a letter requesting more food and medical supplies. With all this activity my supplies were once again falling perilously low. As usual, Diman did not disappoint. He returned with ample quantities of medicine, and the news that several nurses wanted to join our effort in Azad. Apparently they had been so impressed with our work they were overcome with a desire to unite with our team. This latest Pesh Merga I'd sent them turned out to have injuries in both his intestines and pancreas. They had operated immediately, and the patient was reported to be in good condition.

As soon as he'd had time to catch his breath I discussed the matter of a new location for the hospital with Diman. We spent two hours scouting the area until we came across a small valley close to the Daban mountain with hills on three sides. We both knew immediately the area was perfect. It was covered with thick forest and came equipped with a good water supply only two hundred meters away. The Susei garrison couldn't possibly shell it because of its proximity to the Daban mountain, and the forest was so dense that any movement would be undetectable from the air. Within twenty-four hours the local Party official had rounded up twelve men to help us dig in the new wards and treatment rooms we required to be fully functional.

The main building materials were tree branches and thin green stems woven in an artistically creative manner to form walls. The roof was comprised of leafy branches fixed to bamboo poles. Due to a gargantuan team effort working around the clock, we were ready to move patients to the new facility within only two days. We still needed to put finishing touches to the outside theater, complete the second ward, dig trenches (just in case of attack) and arrange the drugs, but it was robust enough to open for business. And just as well – no sooner had we started to move patients when a large group of wounded Pesh Merga arrived on mules. Their injuries were bound in turbans, with apparent fractures supported by wooden splints. A note from the dresser at the front lines explained that due to lack of proper medical supplies adequate first aid had not been possible.

With my medicines still in boxes, and the outside theater yet to be built, I had to think fast. I instructed my people to quickly arrange all the mattresses we had under large trees. In no time we had a makeshift operating room, much to the amazement of a growing crowd of local spectators. At least five of the Pesh Merga were seriously wounded. I dispatched Ali off to the 4th medical section in Pen Jewin with a letter requesting a truck to transport the patients. It was a five-hour walk each way and meantime I had to attend to their injuries with whatever was at my disposal if they were to stand a chance. With only one truck in the area, ferrying everything imaginable back and forth on a daily basis, securing such luxurious transport was a tough call. But I knew these men would never survive the trek on mule, so taking no for an answer simply wasn't an option.

The first Pesh Merga was only twenty-two-years old. He'd been hit in the lower abdomen. He was semi-conscious and fully delirious. He kept heart-wrenchingly calling for his mother while I tried to take his blood pressure. His pulse was rapid and weak, and as usual we were out of blood transfusions and plasma expenders. I made him as comfortable as possible, covered him with blankets, and moved onto the next man.

This Pesh Merga was thirty, and he had a small hole in the middle of his forehead. He was already in a coma with apparent cerebral bleeding. Although there were signs of severe damage to the brain, his heart and circulation systems were functioning normally. However, if I was to save his life I had to operate immediately to remove the foreign body in his head, which appeared to be a shrapnel fragment. I instructed Sherka on the procedure and hurried along to the next patient.

The third case was equally horrific with an injury in the right arm that had opened the entire lower section. His nerves and blood vessels were exposed, and a few tendons had been cut. The wound extended for the full length of his underarm, and it was evident he'd also torn his muscles. Diman was instructed to clean the wound with diluted antiseptic and get the instruments sterile for surgery.

I moved towards the next victim, praying that one day this nightmare would end. The fourth Pesh Merga had an almost fully amputated arm at the elbow. All that could be done was to separate the bone and stitch the wound.

Incredibly the fifth brave soul was a ninety-year-old man! He was amazingly fit; had I met him in the street I wouldn't have judged him to be more than around fifty years old. I was told he was one of the best guides in the area, and battle-hardened from forty years of war. This crusty old soldier had led thirty-seven Pesh Merga to attack the Susei garrison the day before. Sixteen of them were supposed to have moved in and defused the mines, the other twenty-one being the attack force. The old man took the point and inadvertently tripped one of the mines, setting off a chain reaction of explosions that took all sixteen by surprise. After all the battles he'd faced I couldn't allow his life to end this way, not due to the accidental tripping of a landmine.

"This is nothing serious," he told me with determination.

I studied his wounds, wondering what he would consider serious. His left leg and right hand were bound with turbans to bloody pieces of wood. His lips and tongue were blue; the tongue had also split into several pieces. His lower limbs were a compote of flesh, bones, and blood vessels, yet despite all of this he behaved like nothing had happened. Examining him was like peeling an onion. Each new area of his body I uncovered revealed another wound. His son, who was standing resolutely by his side, turned his head away to weep, as though he was ashamed by such an emotional outburst.

"Kora ayba," the old man scowled at his son. "If you keep weeping like a child I will no longer consider you my son."

He was quickly led away – still weeping.

I was unable to amputate his legs without a saw and anesthetic, so I cleaned the wound, removed the bone splinters, and stitched first the tendons, then the muscles, and lastly the skin over the top. All the while the old man was offering encouragement to his wounded comrades, a brave gesture that reduced many of them to tears. The power of the cascading emotions around me was palpable. Even as I treated their wounds I was affected by the sheer weight of it. Surrounded by all this horror I could still be moved by the bravery of a single soul. As I stitched and sewed, I felt the bitter sting of burning tears trickling down my face.

Against all odds this remarkable man survived the procedure and was still alive when I initially put pen to paper to begin writing this manuscript.

The following hours were a blur of broken bones and compound fractures. I lost count of the number of stitches, and the quantity of plaster casts. It was a production line, a macabre factory of human body parts whose fates literary were held between my hands. It was as though I was watching some gruesome other realm theater play out before my eyes.

Finally I received a message that my request for a truck to move the wounded had been granted. It would be with us 'as soon as possible'. "As soon as possible," I repeated to myself. How soon was that? How soon would be soon enough? When would 'soon' be too late? I began to doubt everything – myself, my patient's potential for survival, and most of all – our endurance.

∞∞

Tea and bread! If I live to be three hundred and fifty I doubt I'd care if I never saw tea and bread again. But in Azad in 1974, it was the staple food that kept us alive. As sick as I was of it, I'd hired a woman for twelve pounds a month to bake fresh bread daily. As sick as I was of it, we couldn't afford to ever run out. We supplied the woman with flour, and her family supplied the wood and salt to complete the baking process. Day after day, week after week, month after month, there was always bread.

The truck eventually arrived in Azad in time to successfully transfer my patients to the 4th medical section in Pen Jewin. We weren't five days into our new location and already I felt as though I'd lived there for an eternity. We had three guards patrolling the perimeter of our facility during the day, and between five and eight at night, as well as two in each ward. Somehow we managed to keep our location a secret for the entire duration of our tenure. The fruit trees that so effectively camouflaged us also served as natural decorations. The canopy of our main room was a huge pear tree, around which we simply built four walls. Hundreds of plump, ripe pears dangled overhead like Christmas tree bulbs. I actually found the sight rather comforting. In truth, I was beginning to sense an aura of security around this creatively designed hospital. Nestled among the natural beauty of a land that at times still managed to appear virginal, we had established two wards capable of taking at least twenty-four patients. There was almost nothing to worry about – well nothing aside from the snakes and scorpions.

I didn't like to kill anything, but the thought of having saved a life only to have it snatched away again by a snake bite was obscene. If one or other of us had to die, it would be the snakes. To accomplish that little task I called in the local version of pest control – the Dervish. Dervishes belonged to a rare religious sect that has mastered certain arts incomprehensible to most. Among their astonishing feats was an ability to catch snakes without being bitten by them. Within a few days they'd killed twenty snakes and countless scorpions. By no means did we consider the ground safe to walk on without checking every step, but every creature removed was a threat eliminated. There were, however, still a number of snake and scorpion victims throughout the summer months. The most tragic of these was a middle-aged Pesh Merga who had minor leg and chest wounds.

The man had been placed in a ward comprised of trees, branches and stone. Late one night a sinister reptile slithered into the ward and despite administering immediate injections the man died the following morning from massive internal bleeding. He was the only Pesh Merga fatality in my hospital in over a year. The mortality rate among civilians was far higher, due mainly to the fact that most of those patients were children who weren't brought to see me soon enough. And not all the Pesh Merga I treated survived; some died later in the 4th section medical hospital. But on the whole our survival rate, especially under the grossly inauspicious conditions we worked in, was staggeringly high. Never did we become complacent about death. Each and every life was considered sacred; no one was dispensable. The young, the old and the infirm, they were all precious; so when a father came to me with his eleven-year-old son suffering from a snake bite my heart sank.

"Please, brother doctor, please save my son. We lost his brother last year to a snake bite. He is the only child I have left."

I looked at the boy who was white as paper and stiff as a board and knew it was hopeless. Fiercely destructive emotions swelled in my breast. I felt anger – burning, raging, fires of hell anger against the government's forces, for if not for the war these people wouldn't have been forced to hide out in areas where they were at risk of snakebite.

I took the boy and isolated him from the other patients, so as not to distress them when the inevitable moment arrived. I even managed to get him to drink some chicken soup that night, but by the morning he was gone. I shared every tear and every agonizing moment of grief with his father as the man slowly marched his son away to be buried, his head hanging in bitter defeat.

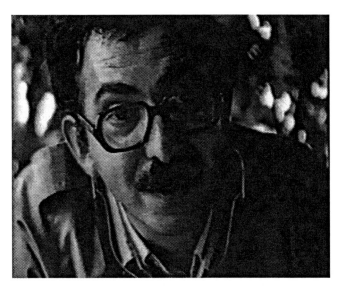

Dr. Med. Albert Gewargis

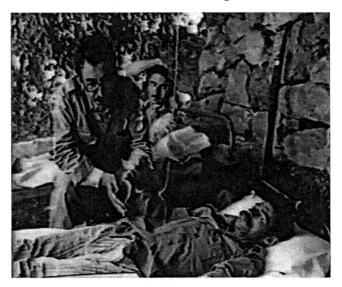

**Brother Doctor with injured Pesh Merga –
men's ward in summer hospital**

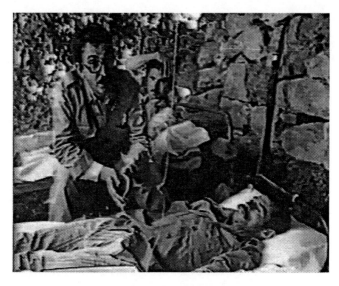

**Brother Doctor in summer hospital (men's ward)
with injured Pesh Merga**

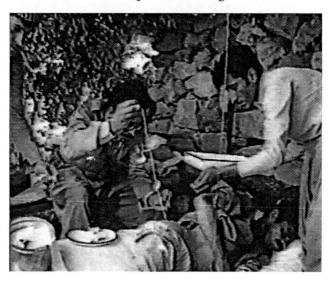

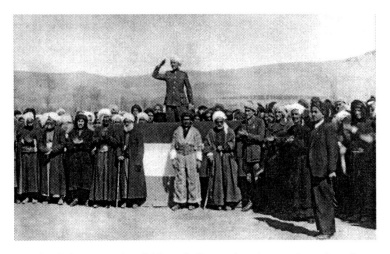

Qazi Mohammed and Mustafa Barzani at the proclamation of
Kurdish Republic of Mahabad, January 22, 1946

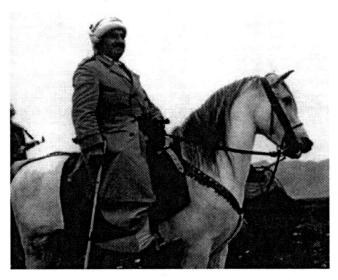

Mustafa Barzani at the proclamation of
Kurdish Republic of Mahabad, January 22, 1946

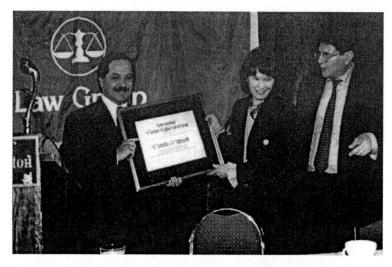

KDP Leader Masoud Barzani receiving an award from International Law Group of Human Rights, presented by Daniella Mitterand, Washington D.C., 1993

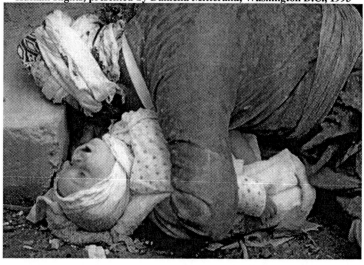

Father and child gassed to death in Halabja, March 1988

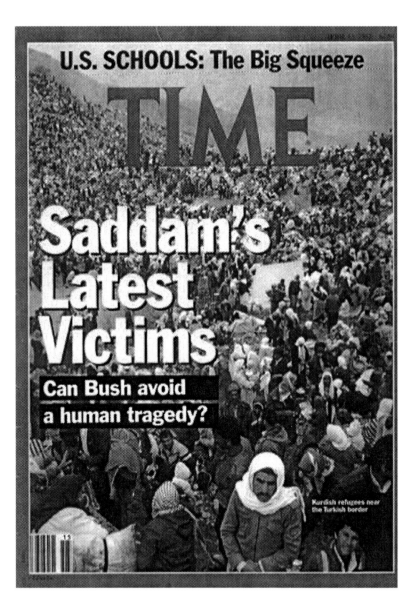

Kurdish exodus of 2 million, April 1991

107

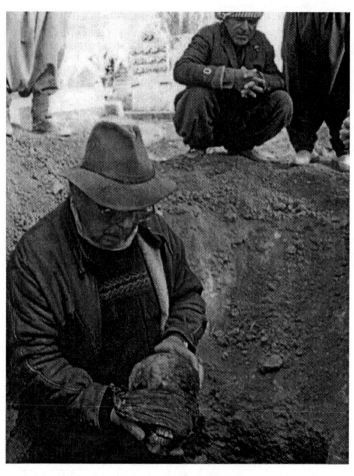

Mass graves of Anfal Campaign discovered, 1991

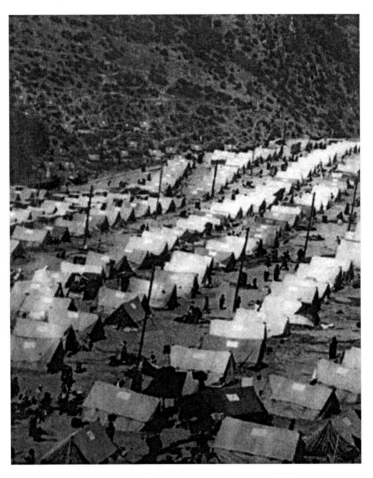

Iraqi Kurdish refugee camp in Iran, 1975

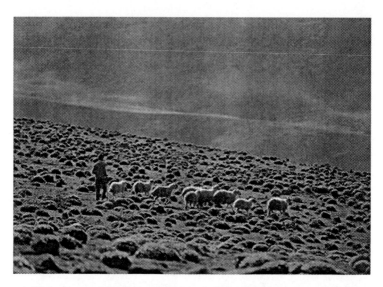

The sweet-smelling purple flowers of the Kurdistan mountains

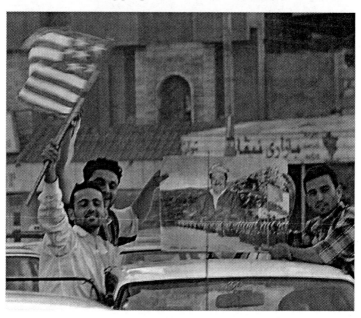

Kurds celebrate the fall of Baghdad with a poster of Barzani

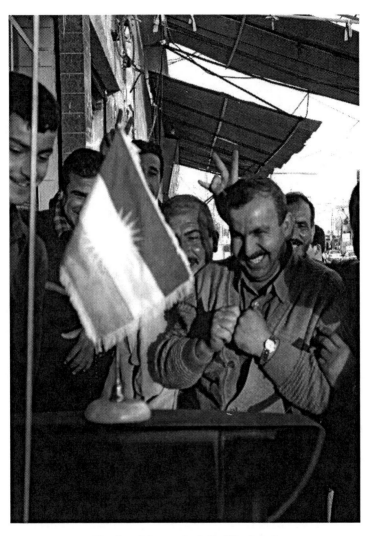

Kurds celebrate the fall of Baghdad

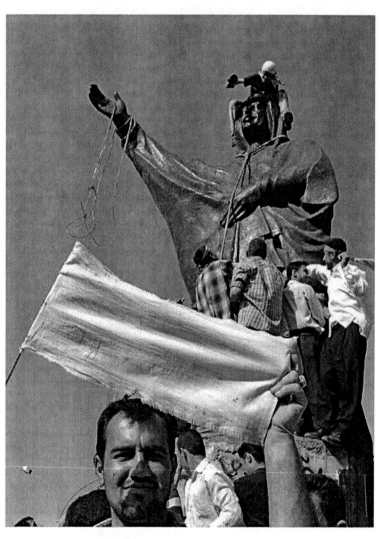

A Kurd in Kirkuk just before Saddam's statue came down

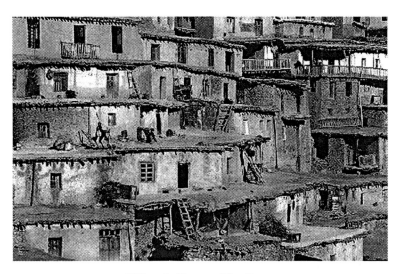

Village in Eastern Kurdistan

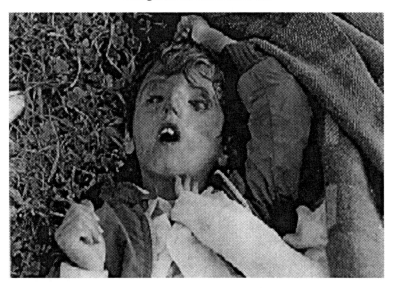

Gassed child with baby

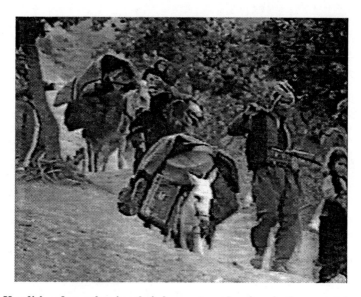

Kurdish refugees leaving their homes to seek refuge in the mountains

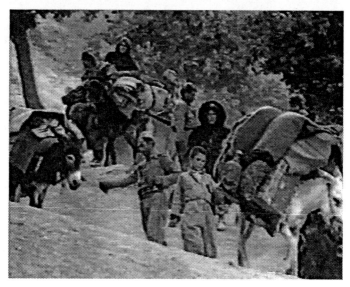

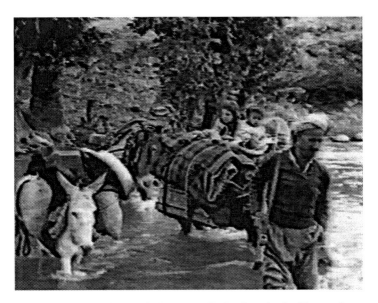

Kurdish families leaving their homes to find refuge in the liberated states

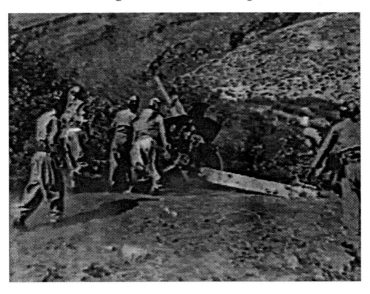

**Pesh Merga hitting a military garrison with primitive artillery
from the peak of the mountains**

115

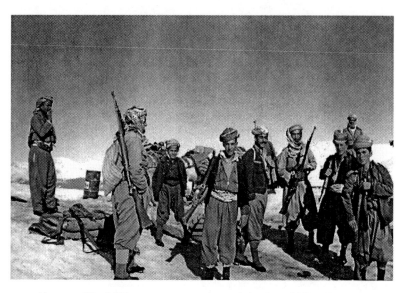

Group of Pesh Merga on mountain peak in the middle of winter

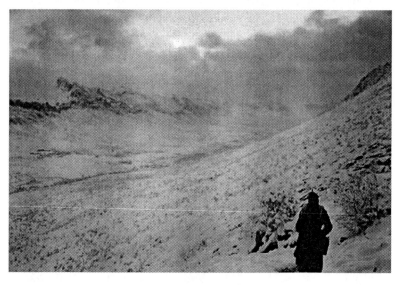

Winter scene outside Azad (Brother Doctor in foreground)

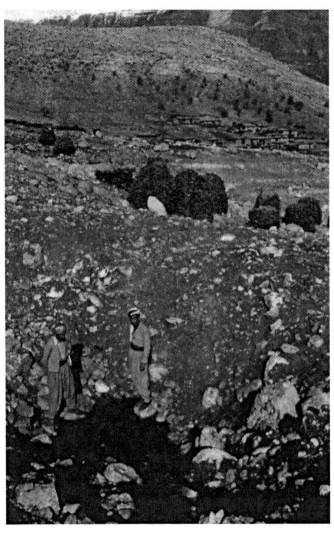

Bomb crater in Azad (part of village in background)

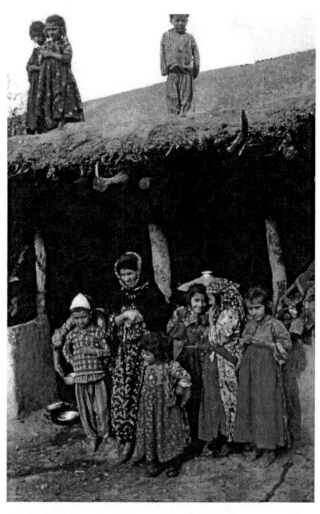

Typical Kurdish family with kids on the roof of the house

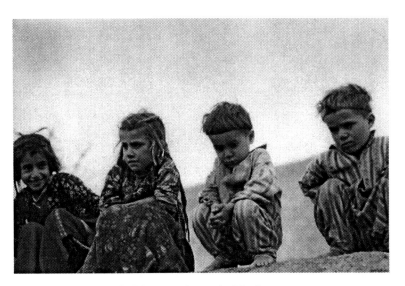

Children on the roof of the house

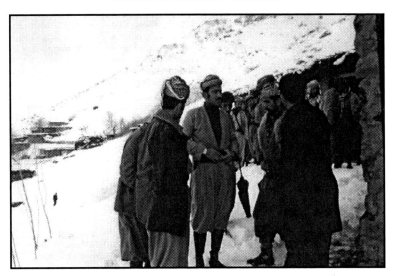

Brother Doctor with Kurdo (second from left)

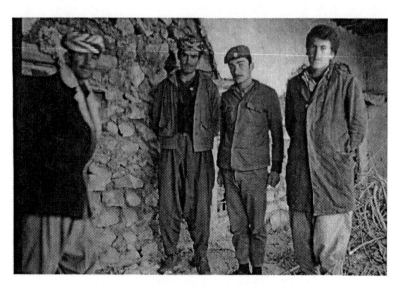

Some imprisoned Iraqi Government soldiers

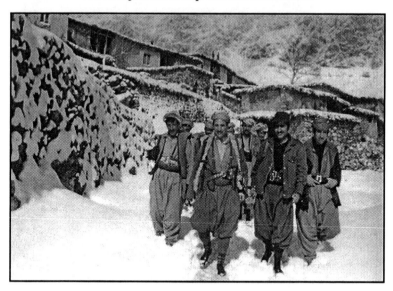

Group of Pesh Merga from battalion three on mission in winter

120

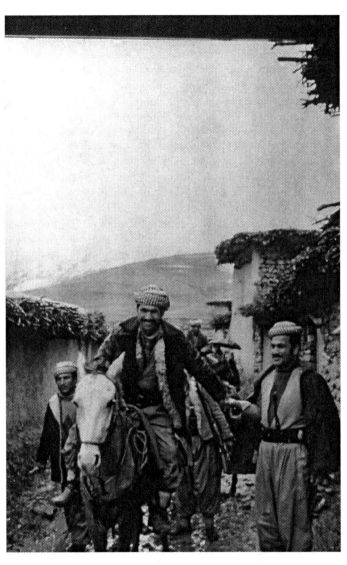

**Commanders of battalion four (Kurdo on the right)
and commander battalion six**

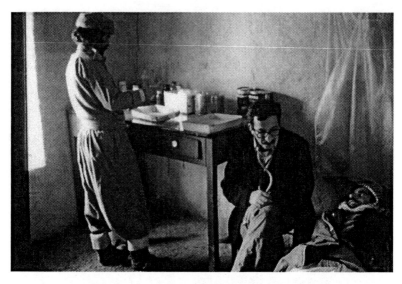

Brother Doctor with severely injured Pesh Merga

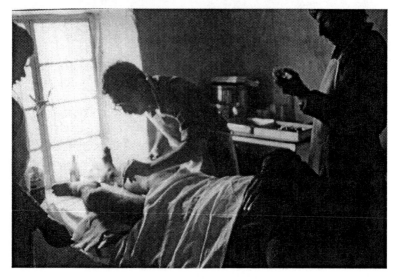

Brother Doctor in operation room (winter hospital)

122

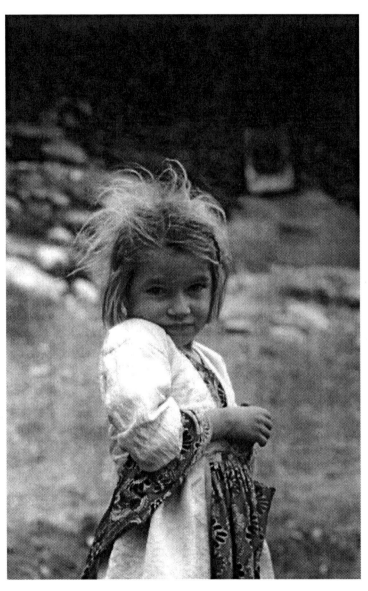

Kurdish child in typical Kurdish dress

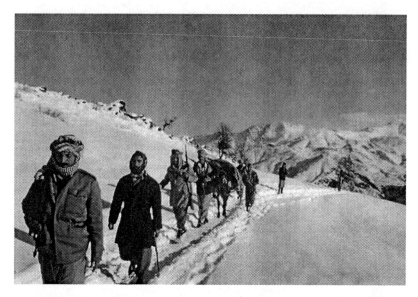

Group of Pesh Merga on a mission on the top of the mountains in the winter

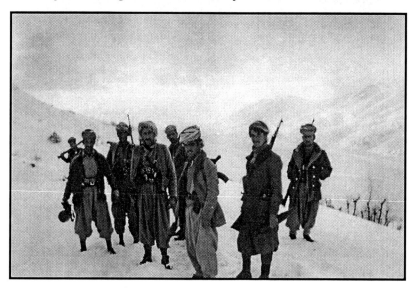

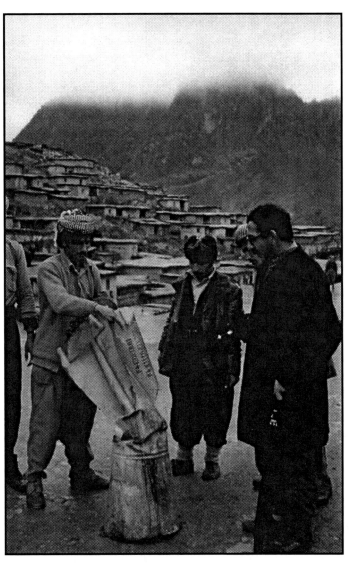

Exploded Russian bomb outside of a village

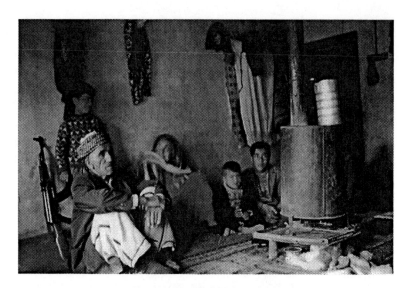

Typical Kurdish living room

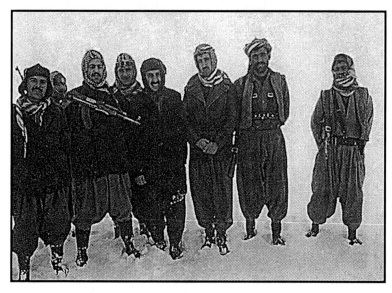

Brother Doctor and Kurdo during the mission on Mt Pira Magron

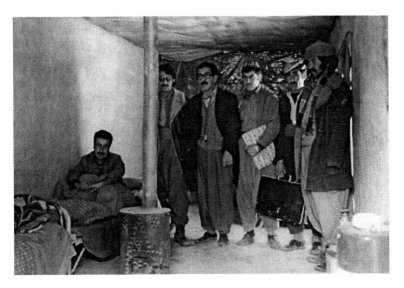

Brother Doctor in front of men's ward with a group of dressers (winter hospital)

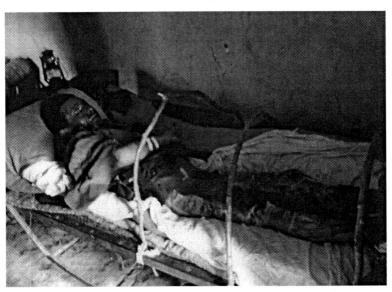

Severely injured napalm civilian casualty

127

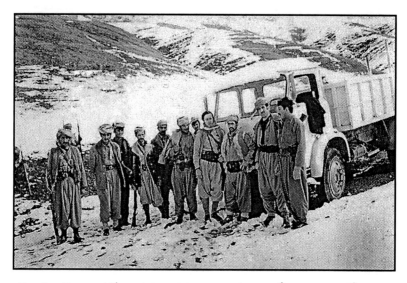

Brother Doctor (1st on right) with commander of 6th battalion (3rd on the right) with the French colleague (4th on the right) after the mission in Sul

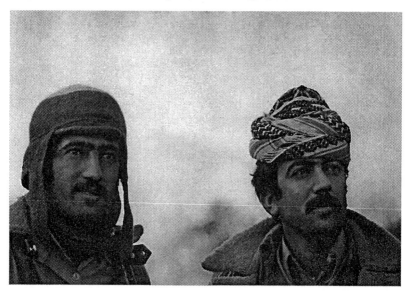

Two young Pesh Merga

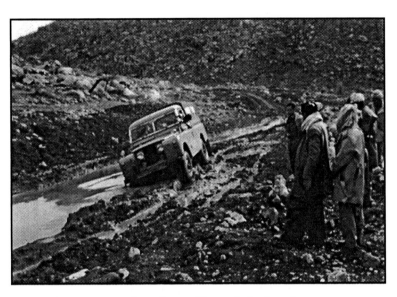

Landrover stuck on the muddy roads in the rainy season

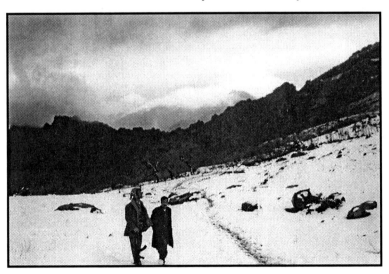

Brother Doctor on a mission

129

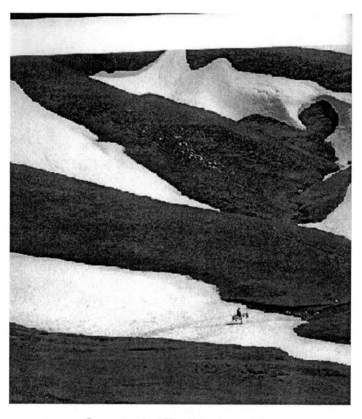

Snow-streaked Kurdistan mountains

CHAPTER TEN

The day after the boy's burial we received some rare good news. The 4th section were so proud of the efforts in my little hospital they were going to send us increased supplies of food and medicine, and more importantly some nurses. The chief surgeon had apparently been amazed at the results we'd been achieving with virtually no resources, and promised to send us anything we asked for provided it was within his ability. I was still seeing no less than two hundred patients a day, but occasionally I managed to sneak away and spend time in my magic garden. Such respite was not without risk as planes could spot me traveling to and fro, but I needed to pretend, at least for a little while, that there was still beauty and freedom in the world.

Our nights were spent around a campfire, drinking tea and listening to the radio – an exercise in futility that we clung to regardless. Night after night we tuned into The Voice of Kurdistan, despite the fact the government's buzzing interference on the frequency made it virtually impossible to understand a single word. Nonetheless, we listened. There were areas in Kurdistan where the programs could be reasonably well received, and as they broadcast reports in Kurdish, Arabic, English, Turkish, and Assyrian the network did a great deal to help keep the peoples' spirit high. The location of the radio station was a closely guarded secret. Throughout the entire war the government never stopped trying to find it, but they never succeeded.

∞∞

Three arduous months slipped by, each moment etched into my memory for a lifetime. My staff complement had grown to around thirty people from a range of backgrounds as diverse as their political leanings. However, we all shared one thing in common – we were bound by a burning desire to help an oppressed people win freedom. I was not the only city-slicker who'd left a comfortable life to endure inconceivable hardship, there were many students and graduates who weren't used to living in the mountains, weren't used to not having meat every day, weren't used to wondering when they'd next be able to bathe, and most of them were certainly not used to washing their own clothes. None of us had lived without electricity before, let alone thought about sleeping on a bed of leaves that was likely home to deadly venomous snakes. We'd read about fighter planes in other wars flying overhead and dropping bombs, but we had no concept of what it was like in reality. Yet no one ran. No one said, "It's too hard." No one said, "It's not my battle." No one was going to give up because everyone believed in what we were doing; we believed stronger, harder, and more fiercely than we'd ever believed in anything in our lives.

Over time we all became numbed to the sound of bombs dropping. We even became a little blasé about the snakes and scorpions, which wasn't clever. The moment you drop your guard is the moment you're going to get stung, as indeed I did. I was lying in bed one night when a scorpion fell out of a tree and onto my chest. Within moments my throat had swollen, making it difficult for me to breathe. All I could think about was what would happen to my hospital if I were to die. I couldn't operate on myself, so I quickly instructed a dresser to get instruments ready with a suitable piece of string tied to a tube in case it would need inserting in my throat. Partially due to the injection I gave myself, and partially due to a gritty resolve that it was far too inconvenient for me to die, I survived the experience relatively unscathed.

I thought I'd seen it all.

I was wrong.

Soon I would be called to Schwan to deal with a sudden outbreak of measles that had already killed over one hundred children in that area alone. But before that day arrived I treated a case that will live with me forever.

A sixteen-year-old girl from Askar, newly married with a baby, was out washing dishes in the well when an air raid struck. A vast piece from one of the rockets hit the girl squarely in the chest and upper arm. With awe-inspiring bravery, and perhaps a touch of maternal instinct, she managed to throw her infant away from the blast. She was rewarded by receiving the full brunt of the attack herself. The young girl was in such bad shape that her husband refused to take her to the hospital in Azad; it took considerable persuasion by her mother and a Party official to change his mind.

She was wrapped tightly in a blanket and put in a coffin tied to a mule for the eight-hour journey. When she was ultimately placed on my operating table I thought she was already dead. Her pulse and blood pressure were unregisterable. I think I was biting my bottom lip, believing it was too late, when she made a weak crying noise. The devoted mother was in such a state of shock she didn't seem to be feeling any pain, but if I was going to save her life I needed to work fast – and I needed blood. Everyone was willing to donate, but no one present was the right blood type.

The three dressers working with me were all O+, which was the closest match I was likely to get to the girl's B+. Without losing a moment I took a pint from each of them, feeling a little like a Middle-Eastern Count Dracula. We boiled our primitive and incomplete instruments and poured concentrated antiseptic over them. The dressers took twenty minutes to clean out the wounds as they were clogged with mud and grease from the bombing site. As I scrubbed, it occurred to me that even if I successfully treated her wounds, she was still likely to die from tetanus.

Her right breast was cut into two halves. Her upper right arm was completely shattered. The underarm was open with nerves and blood vessels exposed. The major blood vessels were all destroyed. Her arm was irreparable. The fingers were dark blue and had an offensive odor wafting from them indicating to me that the limb was already quite dead. I gave her a sedative, even though she was apparently feeling

133

no pain, and set to work amputating the arm – a procedure I'd never undertaken before. Operating by only the light of an oil lamp, without a bone saw, I had to use pliers to cut and straighten the bone and stitch the massive wound with regular thread. There was just enough catgut on hand to stitch and tie the muscles and vessels. When I next looked at the clock, three hours had slipped past.

Exhausted, numb, perhaps a little in shock myself, I took her blood pressure and pulse again. Her pulse was rapid but steady. It was encouraging, even though the thought of tetanus wasn't far from my mind. Her amputated arm was washed, wrapped in a white cloth and buried according to religious custom, while I headed to the kitchen to discuss the case with my colleagues.

It took many weeks, but eventually the girl was strong enough to be taken by mule to a Kurdish hospital just across the border in Iran. There was a chance she could be fitted with an artificial arm in this facility, although I doubted having a new limb would do anything to ease her troubled mind. The trauma she'd endured was unimaginable to most. Her innocent young mind had been plunged into a world of darkness with no passageways back towards the light. Not a night went by that she wasn't plagued with nightmares, waking in a cold sweat, running for her life from a foe more terrifying than the blackest monsters of myth and legend.

I watched her leave allowing myself a moment of self-indulgent reflection – what would life have in store for her now she was mutilated in both mind and body? Did the government ever stop to think, even for an instant, about the twisted malevolence they perpetrated on their fellow human beings? It was a ridiculous rhetorical question. Evil has no conscience.

∞∞

In Schwan the measles epidemic was raging. Most of the dressers in the area were old timers who liked to work independently with the Pesh Merga, leaving little time for sick civilians. As requested, Darwish, two villagers, and two mules loaded with medicines accompanied me to the area. Our first stop was at the 4th battalion headquarters, where I requested some Pesh Merga to escort us through the hot spots of the journey. The most dangerous sector was crossing the main highway near the Susei garrison. This was a popular spot for nighttime ambushes by both sides. The commander told us he'd assign five Pesh Merga to our group, and for part of the way he'd travel with us himself as he had a patrolling mission towards Surdash.

We had to wait until the very dead of night before continuing the journey, as the road between Schwan and Surdash was both very flat and very close to the government's troops. Fortunately the night sky was moonless; however disappearing under the cover of darkness did nothing to disguise any sound we might make. I heard every crunch underfoot as we cautiously progressed, especially the firm footsteps of the confident Pesh Merga. At times we came within ten meters of the government outposts before arriving on the outskirts of Surdash. Covered behind a hill our group split in two, the commander and his Pesh Merga going one way, and the medical team with our Pesh Merga scouts heading another. The silent tension was overwhelming, furtive glances occasionally being exchanged among my nervous medical crew.

"Stop or I'll shoot," one of our Pesh Merga scouts suddenly shouted.

"Don't shoot your own," someone hissed back from the darkness.

Gradually faces belonging to the footsteps our scout had heard emerged from the black surrounds; a man and his wife accompanied by their infant and two mules.

"I'm sorry," the scout huffed.

"You are right to be wary," the man told him. "There are rumors of an ambush with tanks at the main crossing point."

"There always are," the Pesh Merga replied dispassionately.

The man mumbled under his breath about the Pesh Merga's indifference and continued on his way. Not ten minutes passed before his grim prediction proved true. Heavy firing started from the military outposts surrounding Surdash. It sounded like RBG 7 and Doshka fire interrupted by intensive automatic weapons. From what we could tell the assault was coming from three separate directions. The forces in Surdash immediately switched on their observation lights, flooding

135

the area with dazzling beams that gave the illusion of high noon. Up ahead we heard a group of people hidden behind some rocks engaged in heated argument. Darwish and a Pesh Merga went to investigate.

"They are villagers, and they say the tanks are on the highway again," Darwish explained to me moments later. Turning firmly towards the Pesh Merga he added, "We can't risk the life of brother doctor, we have to turn back."

"Brother doctor can cross after we have crossed and the street is cleared," the Pesh Merga told him simply.

"I agree," I added. "But the medicines have to be kept safe at all costs. The two villagers should wait until last with the mules. If there's any sign of trouble they must return."

"But we welcome death with you, brother doctor," one of the villagers piped up.

I gazed at them with sad, proud eyes. It was obvious none of us were turning back, so I took a deep breath and followed the Pesh Merga's path into the fray. My heart was pounding so hard I thought it might actually leap out of my chest. We crossed a stream and headed towards a narrow muddy path through some trees, hoping and praying we would escape unwanted attention. My ears pricked to the sound of the Pesh Merga cocking their rifles as we approached the highway. It was three meters wide and flat as a pancake. I froze on the spot, looking left and right and left again just as I'd been taught to do when crossing the road as a boy. We'd calculated that the Susei garrison was shelling the surrounding villages at thirty minute intervals – that was our window of opportunity to move.

Approaching another flooded river with no bridge we were forced to wade waist-deep across strong currents towards Awahlahen. It must have been around midnight when we reached the outskirts of this village heading straight for the mosque. Mosques were frequently used by the Pesh Merga during the war; they provided shelter and adequate washing facilities, usually in the form of a large basin of running water. Of course they also provided a place to offer prayers, but the army's forces were wise to this. No longer was anyone safe inside a mosque. Nothing was sacred in war-torn Iraq.

Rather than head inside we settled in a big yard outside the mosque, from where we could hear water flowing in the basin. All among us were devilishly tired, horribly hungry and disgustingly dirty. I took my shoes off and threw myself into the basin to bathe while Darwish shared out a few tomatoes and some bread for our exhausted crew. This humble repast did little to quench our ravenous appetites. Poor Darwish, he was so determined to find us something else to eat that he turned on his flashlight to see what else he could find.

"For God's sake, turn out that light," one of the Pesh Merga hissed – but it was too late. Within seconds an artillery shell hit around twenty meters in front of the mosque. We all flung ourselves on the ground as a second, third, and fourth shell hit the area. Mules started baying, dogs started barking, and I found myself again wondering if this was where it was all going to end.

It seemed an eternity, but it was probably only a few moments before the army apparently lost interest in bombing us. A little shaken I found my shoes and tried to put them back on. They wouldn't fit! On closer inspection I saw that my feet had become dreadfully swollen. I remember glancing around to see if anyone had noticed my predicament before deciding they would *have* to fit. The Pesh Merga were eager to move on once our position had been compromised, and it was a three-hour walk to our next stop, the village of Kalascher. Swollen feet were not a primary consideration in the scheme of things.

The route, as usual, was an arduous one. We had a one-hour climb up a mountain, in the dark, over a rough and narrow road. It was decided the mules would go first as once they'd made a journey they could find their way again even if it was pitch black. One of the villagers who owned one of these trusty steeds stopped and had a few words with him before we commenced our climb. I couldn't help but be touched by the soft and soothing tone he took with this sturdy animal, it was as though he was speaking to a baby.

Sure enough the mules led the way up the eighty-degree incline until we reached the summit.

"Oh my," I gasped, gazing around the landscape. There, in the distant vast panorama below us, I could see the everlasting fires of Baba Kurgur, reputed to have been burning since the days of Nebuchadnezzar. An entire city was bathed in a reddish gold light that resembled a perpetual sunrise. It was truly breathtaking, but it left me with one inescapable thought – DAMN OIL! If it wasn't for oil we might have been free many years ago.

Of course what goes up must come down again, and our descent down the mountain was quite terrifying, on a path only a few feet wide with a sheer drop of hundreds of meters into a rocky valley below. Even the mules were having trouble, and my poor feet positively wanted to disown me! Although I tried to put on a brave face, the Pesh Merga could see I was shaky. One of them silently took up position on my outside for the rest of the way. Such very brave and noble men.

It was somewhere between three and four in the morning when we arrived at Kala Scher, the headquarters of the 2nd battalion of the Ruzgari Brigade. The village was almost deserted with only four families remaining, but those families were known for their hospitality towards the Pesh Merga. Even though it was the holy festival of Ramadan, during which fasting was observed from sunrise to sunset for a full month, fortunately the sun had not yet risen. Darwish knocked at a door, hoping we'd find a friendly face on the other side. The sound of shuffling footsteps approached and the door creaked slowly open. An old woman looked us up and down, immediately recognizing Pesh Merga.

"Be kar bin farmo," she cheered, meaning roughly, 'You are welcome'.

The mules were unloaded, we were shown to a guest room, and gallons of sweet tea were served while food was prepared. This presented an opportunity to examine my poor feet. I discovered they were not only swollen but bleeding and blistered as well. I sighed with a heavy resolve knowing the journey was far from over, and wondering how I'd withstand the rest of it.

With gluttonous gusto we devoured all the yogurt and fried bread the woman could give us. I dare say our table manners left something to be desired, but having eaten virtually nothing in twenty-four hours we didn't care.

With his belly full, one of the Pesh Merga turned to me. "Brother doctor, may we have permission to leave now?"

"But you haven't rested," I responded in slight shock.

"We have another twenty-four hours of walking ahead," he explained. "There is no time to rest."

Truly if I could have bottled the stamina of these men I would have never needed any other form of medicine. They weren't showing even the slightest sign of fatigue. Sometimes I wondered if they were really robots, but then I reminded myself of the blood I'd seen spilled. I wanted to give each and every one of them a medal for their bravery. Such very remarkable men.

The next morning my feet were still in terrible shape. On noticing my condition our host offered me a pair of rubber shoes, undoubtedly the most practical footwear in Kurdistan. Although my next destination was close by, it was heavenly to have feet that were at least a little happier. The 2nd battalion's headquarters was only a half hour's walk away, situated deep in a valley where their tents were effectively camouflaged by nut trees. They'd established an impressive system for supplying fresh cool water to their hideout from a five hundred meter tube attached to a nearby well. The inventiveness of these people never ceased to amaze me. Anwar, their chief dresser, came running out to greet us the moment we arrived, taking me immediately to the dispensary in a small cave where forty people were already waiting to see me. They had no medicines whatsoever; they hadn't even been paid in over three months. Although no one complained about the lack of wages, operating on the front lines with no bandages, penicillin, anti-tetanus, pain killers or stitching silk was impossible.

I saw over one hundred patients that day, most of them children suffering from malnutrition and acute diarrhea with up to ten percent fluid depletion. Thrown into the mix were a few severe cases of measles, bronchitis, pneumonia, and two suspected cases of encephalitis. The worst of these was a thirteen-year-old boy who came to see me with his seventy-year-old grandfather, who was also sick. I was advised that the child's father was already dead. Apparently they lived in a neighboring village where some Pesh Merga had told them that 'doctor gawra' (big doctor) was coming to town. The boy was dry, toxic and weak with a temperature of 40oC. I tried without success to convince the old man to send the boy to the hospital in Azad for treatment, but he wouldn't be parted from him for a moment – a fact that ultimately and tragically almost certainly led to the boy's death.

That evening I divided half of the medicine I had between the 1st, 2nd, and 5th battalions, and took the remaining half with us on the rest of our journey. We started for the village of Gop Tapa with a Pesh Merga from the 2nd battalion, calculating we should be there in five hours if all went well. There was only one valley to cross and one mountain to climb, the rest of the terrain was flat. The route took us through a beautiful oasis of fruit trees and babbling brooks. Quietly I envied their tranquility and perfection, wondering why mankind couldn't emulate such a peaceful existence.

The pain in my feet had become unbearable. Although I didn't like to ride the mules, I was left with no other choice. I realized that crossing flat land on mule back made me an easy target, but fortunately the next air raid held off until after I'd dismounted to rest at a small deserted settlement. Their target on this occasion was the 2nd battalion headquarters and the villages surrounding Sargelow, which was uncomfortably close. We watched as the planes expertly maneuvered behind the nearby mountains, unable to do anything but gaze with profound sadness as enormous explosions echoed throughout the land. An unwelcome and hideous feeling of impotence crawled through my veins.

"We have to go," one of the Pesh Merga told me.

I ached with a longing to help the wounded we knew would be suffering in Sargelow, but the cold fact of the matter was we were already behind schedule, and the people in Gobtapa needed my assistance more desperately.

Omar, the chief dresser of Gobtapa, restlessly awaited our arrival in the mosque. I wasn't allowed to relax for an instant after the arduous journey we'd undertaken.

"There's a woman who's very sick, brother doctor," Omar told me. "You must come at once."

Dutifully I followed the dresser to a young woman's home. She was pale as toothpaste and in a state of shock. When I lifted the blanket I was sickened to see she was also lying in a pool of blood.

"Is she pregnant?" I asked the lady attending to her.

"She delivered a dead baby this morning. I couldn't get the placenta out."

It had become an all too familiar sight.

Water was boiled, soap was procured, and the men were all asked to leave. The woman had a complete placenta adhesion, which I removed manually with careful sawing-like movements. An injection of a uterus-contracting drug arrested the bleeding, but Omar had been right – there hadn't been a minute to lose.

Anger once again began to swell in my breast.

"Why didn't you do anything to try and help her?" I asked Omar afterwards.

"I did not know what to do," he told me simply.

I sighed heavily, determined that before I left this village every dresser would understand what caused bleeding in pregnancy and in future they would know how to deal with it. Omar hurriedly scribbled notes in a little book as I barked out a précised course in the finer points of bush gynecology. Meanwhile my patient was improving, but she needed blood. Tests revealed that her husband was the only suitable donor.

"But I cannot give blood to a woman," he gasped, when I suggested the notion. "It would be shameful. My father would never allow it."

His sister loomed up beside him with a disapproving scowl. "I will give blood, brother doctor," she offered.

"That's very generous of you, but you're not the right blood type."

She turned towards her brother once more, her brow furrowed with fury. "If you do not give blood to your wife and she dies you will have to find three hundred pounds to marry another woman to care for your children."

The husband grimaced back at this sister, but reluctantly agreed that the lesser of two evils was apparently to give blood. I did love these people, but at times I just couldn't understand how they could rationalize a faith that allowed their loved ones to die rather than risk what they saw as dishonor and shame. However, I wasn't about to facilitate a fundamental shift in philosophical thinking during my brief tenure, and anyway I still had to deal with the measles epidemic that had brought me to this region.

141

On approaching Ahmed, the local Party official, a sudden chill swept through me as though a prophetic demon of death was laughing at our efforts. The wind seemed to whisper, "Beat you." When I looked into Ahmed's eyes I could see immediately it was true.

"If only you'd arrived here three days ago," he said sadly.

I don't remember what he said after that, I only remember being led towards the village cemetery.

Wicked whisperings in the wind whisked around me as my gaze stretched across the burial ground. I stood there for what felt like endless excruciating eons gawping at so many tiny and freshly dug graves.

"Seventy children aged between two and eleven died in the last three days," he told me solemnly. "It is almost all the children in the village."

Gritting my teeth and wiping a futile tear from my eye I turned to the official. "Was there nothing you could have done?"

"We've had no supplies for nearly three months. No medicine. What could we do?"

"Well, we have medicine now. Show me where I can set up a hospital facility."

Perhaps ironically the chosen location for my latest hospital was the deserted school. With drone-like efficiency we set about the task of establishing yet another temple of medicine where I hoped to work miracles on the few survivors who remained. No sooner had we begun the procedure when the bitter sound of bomber planes screeched overhead once more.

"They're going to bomb Askar again," Omar and Ahmed said almost as one.

From our close proximity we could clearly see four bombs plummet onto the tiny and already battle-scarred village. A heartbeat later the familiar explosions resonated for miles around, followed by storm clouds of black smoke billowing in the wind that so persistently mocked my efforts.

"There will be injured in Askar," I said gloomily. "Please bring them to me."

I thought of Sabria, the sixteen-year-old injured woman. Before leaving Azad to come here she had asked me how her child was doing. I asked Hama to go to her home to find out. When Hama returned he told me that the baby had died in the same bombing incident where Sabria got injured. Such memories haunt me to this day.

Omar left immediately with a small bag of medicine, a villager, and a mule.

"This building will not be enough," I told Ahmed.

He nodded and took me to the outskirts of the village where there was a row of deserted houses.

"Will this do?" he asked.

I peered inside to discover, to my dismay, that these homes had once again been used as a refuge for animals. They were filthy. I glanced accusingly at Ahmed.

"We will supply people to help clean," he said simply, obviously understanding my unspoken rebuke.

Exhaustion was developing a new meaning for me. To be merely exhausted was almost exultation. The weariness I experienced of mind, body, and soul had no human word to describe it. Even the means by which food was obtained in this village was disgusting to my sensibilities. A few grams of explosive powder extracted from unexploded bombs were put in a glass bottle, a fuse was attached and lit, and the device was tossed into the river. Moments later hundreds of fish appeared on their backs. It was brutal, but without any other source of protein these fish were the difference between life and death. The villagers procured their haul by whatever means was at their disposal, and I had no choice but to eat the fish.

It was eleven at night before Omar returned with five wounded. Three people had been killed instantly, one of them a twelve-year-old girl who had literally been blown into pieces that splattered across the area. Eighteen houses had been completely destroyed.

"We'll need beds," I said matter-of-factly to Ahmed.

The homes had been well-cleaned by this time. With medicines and beds we were as functional as we were likely to be for my first patient. She was a thirty-six-year-old woman, who was semi-conscious with a skull fracture and vomiting frequently. Alongside her was a forty-five-year-old man with an almost totally shattered knee joint and multiple face and chest injuries. The third casualty was an eighteen-year-old boy with a femur shaft fracture. He particularly stands out in my memory because he was so afraid he'd rather hide out in a cave than remain with us. I couldn't find it within myself to argue with him for I knew as well as he did that our buildings could easily be the target of the next air raid.

I treated the skull fracture first. Without subjecting the reader to further gore – it was a mess. By the time I finished treating all the injured it was one in the morning, and still there was a great deal of work to do to prepare for patients who would be on my doorstep come sun up.

∞∞

En route to the makeshift hospital the next morning I stopped in to check on the placenta retention patient. She had a slight fever and a headache, but the bleeding had stopped and overall she was progressing well. I smiled at her kindly, impressed by her improvement. In reply she grabbed my hand.

"Brother doctor," she said in a weak voice. "I am going to make you a saint."

"Actually you have your husband to thank," I told her.

She looked at me with quizzical eyes.

"He donated the blood that saved your life," I explained.

She turned and looked at her husband, bursting into tears (which I took to be a sign of gratitude). No time to ponder. I had to get to my latest hospital.

Back at the facility over two hundred patients were already waiting, each mother accompanied my multiple sick children. The vision of seventy little graves burned blindingly in my mind as I looked at the sea of sad faces. It would have been unthinkable to give them anything less than everything I had – these people had suffered enough. I worked from 8:00am until 2:30pm, at which point I took a break for a quick lunch – of fish. There was no shortage of fish after six dynamite bombs had been exploded. Fried fish, smoked fish, boiled fish – fish, fish, fish!

144

The fish dish concluded I returned to my surgery, somewhat surprised to see only seventy-five patients. Had I offended someone?

"The people in the surrounding villages have not all arrived yet," Ahmed explained. "There will be more tomorrow."

He wasn't joking. The next morning there were five hundred people waiting to see me! Considering the village of Gobtapa had a total population of three hundred, I treated two and a half thousand patients in five days! Needless to say this more than exhausted my medical supplies – not to mention my mind and my body. I had to get back to Azad as quickly as possible. The dressers in this village had benefited from my visit by receiving medical training that was nothing short of an initiation by fire, but they needed medicines to continue the work. And they weren't alone. I'd received a message from the Party official in Awahlahen to advise that the measles epidemic had spread to that village too. I found myself wondering if there was enough medicine in the whole world to deal with the problems in Kurdistan.

And still the heartache continued. As I was leaving Gobtapa, Ahmed came to me with information that hundreds more patients were flooding across the nearby mountains to see me, many of them bringing children sick with measles. All I could do was promise I would send another mission as soon as I returned to Azad, but in my heart I knew for many of them it would already be too late. In truth it was a health hazard for this many people to be gathered in one place, disease aside. Large crowds always attracted the attention of the army, and that was invariably followed by a volley of mortar fire. However, trying to stop them coming was akin to King Canute trying to hold back the ocean with a broom.

Ahmed and a few of the villagers escorted us to the outskirts of their domain. As I passed by the cemetery I gazed once more on the seventy tiny graves – so fresh, so small, so tragic.

CHAPTER ELEVEN

The expedition back to Azad was full of the usual trials and tribulations, and the usual hoards of sick and injured at each stop requiring attention. Infrequently there were moments of beauty that reminded me what we were fighting for: the simple beauty of resting under a walnut tree, the vineyards so heavily laden with ripe grapes that I think even the mules had their fill, and most astonishingly of all, I returned to Azad to discover a *female* nurse!

Nurses had often expressed a desire to help with my frontier administrations, but the idea of having a woman working alongside men in this strictly Muslim village seemed unthinkable. Aside from that, I wanted to know how the heck she got there! I really wanted to know... I real ... I really needed some sleep. The problem could wait until tomorrow.

The following day I surprised myself by not waking until four in the afternoon. The first thing I did was call the nurse. All I could think of was that having an unmarried woman working among twenty hot-blooded men was a recipe for disaster.

"Good afternoon, doctor," she said politely.

"Hello, Laila. Please, sit down."

She did.

"I was a little surprised to find you here. When did you arrive?" I asked evenly.

"Three days ago on a medical mission with the chief doctor of the Movement."

"Why didn't you return with him?"

"Because I wanted to stay and work here," she said simply.

"But it's very difficult to live here. We're frequently bombed, especially at this time of year, and the Susei garrison often shells us several times throughout the night."

"I know. But, doctor, I've been thinking about this for a long time, and I strongly believe the best thing I can do for my people is to remain at the front. I've heard a great deal about your hospital. Please don't send me back."

"But where will you stay? Living in the village is impossible, and we don't have a room for you here. There's not even a bath."

"Don't worry, doctor. I've lived under such conditions before. I'll manage."

I studied her body language and looked firmly into her eyes as she spoke. I could see there was no dissuading her. I did desperately need an experienced nurse, and to add gilding to the deal she also informed me she was an experienced midwife. There was no question that I could use one of those!

"Okay," I finally admitted defeat. "You can stay. But don't you come crying to me every day about the conditions!"

"Doctor," she laughed. "If you see me crying just once, you can send me away immediately."

Well, that seemed to be an end to the debate. We had some tea, discussed the situation in Pen Jewin, and I accompanied her over to the women's ward to see what she'd accomplished in my absence.

There was nothing like a woman's touch!

The ward was organized with fresh bed linen, a small table for injection material, a stove, and some instruments. The corner was neatly arranged around a table stacked with dishes, water, and glasses. I was very impressed. My little frontier outpost was now equipped with an excellent lab technician, a very good dentist, some of the best dressers in the area, and Allah preserve us – a nurse! For the first time I felt things might just be about to improve. We even had good stocks of medicine.

A woman in a nearby village agreed to join us, both to help attend to patients and to be a companion to Laila. A small room was built for them adjacent to the women's ward, and a guard permanently positioned close by.

147

∞∞

The month of August rolled unerringly towards us with no let up in hostilities. I saw things time and again that no decent soul should ever have to see. Up until now all of my patients had been 'my' people. Midsummer brought a change to that state of affairs when a wounded army soldier was presented to me for treatment. He'd been caught in an ambush set by the Pesh Merga while he was driving a truck on the main highway three kilometers from the Susei garrison. The truck had been completely destroyed, and the soldier dragged out of the wreckage with multiple lacerations all over his body.

"Please don't kill me," he begged, raising his bleeding arms.

An educated Pesh Merga who spoke Arabic replied stonily, "We don't kill prisoners."

Unlike many instances that were reversed, the Kurdish Movement treated all prisoners of war according to the Geneva Convention. They were given food, shelter, and even a daily financial allowance. For most of them, imprisonment meant a better life than that which they'd come from.

I unraveled the wounded soldier from his bloodied turban bandages to assess the damage.

"Where do you come from?" I asked in Arabic.

"Omarha, in Southern Iraq."

"Ah, I know the area."

"You are not Kurd?"

"I'm Iraqi, and a human being, as are we all."

He looked a little uncertain; hardly surprising given the propaganda I knew their troops were fed by the lying fascist regime in Baghdad. I persisted with conversation, learning he was twenty-six years-old and the father of three children.

"Believe me, doctor, I was forced to stay in the army. Two years ago I was supposed to be released from service, but they didn't let me go home. I am against the war. I hate the Ba'ath."

Of course he would have said that in his present surroundings, but the soulfulness of his eyes indicated to me he was telling the truth.

148

"You don't have to be afraid here," I told him softly. "We are all Iraqis here, fighting against a fascist government so we may all be free one day."

"What's going to happen to me?" he asked in almost a whisper.

"You don't need to worry about a thing," I assured him, looking at the puncture wounds that dotted his entire body.

Fortunately none of his wounds were serious. There were no fractures and no nerve damage; in fact all the lacerations were quite effectively treated with antiseptic. Once he was cleaned up and almost mummified in bandages, he was placed in the men's ward with a close guard. Night after night this tormented soul would wake screaming, "Don't kill me! I'm innocent!" The night guards would give him a glass of water and try to calm him down, but invariably the dresser had to give him an extra sedative.

I was quite certain he wouldn't try and escape. For one thing, he was hardly capable of standing, let alone walking or running. For another, the entire area was swarming with Pesh Merga, so any attempt to escape would have meant certain death. But most of all, we treated him very well. He was given all the food he needed, all the cigarettes he wanted, and extra tea every day. As soon as he was able to walk he was also given new clothes.

When the Brigade commander visited to inspect my hospital and came across the Iraqi soldier, the injured man instantly leapt to his feet.

"Remain seated, my son," the commander said kindly in Arabic. "This is not the army here. Although," he added proudly, "I am an infantry major general." He paused for a moment to let that sink in. "Where are you from?"

"From Omarha, sir," the soldier replied formally.

"Has your treatment been good?"

"Very good, sir. Thank you, sir."

"We are all brothers here, son. You should feel at home. If you have any wishes, tell them to brother doctor. We will do our best to make your stay here comfortable."

"Yes, sir. Thank you, sir." He paused. "Sir?"

"What is it?"

"What will happen to me after I'm released from hospital? Will I be able to go back to my family? Will I be able to see my children...?" The word 'children' trailed on his lips, tears beginning to form in his eyes.

"This is war, my son," the commander said firmly. "As soon as the war is over you can go in peace to your family. Until then, you'll have to remain with us."

"Where will I stay, sir?"

"In the hospital until you are well, then you'll be transferred to an area where hundreds of soldiers are housed. If you have any message or letters to your family we will be glad to send them for you."

The wounded soldier fell silent.

Under our watchful eye, our Iraqi brother recovered quickly and was in due course sent to the Brigade headquarters prison where I decided to pay him a visit. I found him playing dominos with some of the other prisoners, looking quite relaxed. When he spotted me he left the game and rushed towards me, hugging and kissing me as though we were old friends.

"How are you feeling?" I asked.

"I am well, thank you."

Prison was still prison, but if one had to be in prison, one could certainly be in worse places. The inmates were allowed plenty of time in the fresh air of the surrounding fields, and given plenty to keep their minds occupied as the war went on – and on – and winter once again approached.

The leafy canopies of our summer hospital would not suffice once the unrelenting rains of winter commenced again. It was time to move. Just as I'd managed to organize things almost perfectly, we had to dismantle the whole operation and look for a new location. Wandering into the kitchen, Diman immediately picked up on my mood.

"Kaka doctor," ('kaka' means 'brother'). "Kaka doctor, you look as though there's something on your mind."

"You're right. I've been thinking about winter. It's only three months away, and we can't possibly stay where we are now."

"I know," Diman said thoughtfully. "I've been wondering what we're going to do. We can't move back to the school building."

"That's true," I agreed. "It's too small and besides it's an easy target for the army. But from what everyone's been telling me, we'll be completely cut off from the outside world for over four months. It will be impossible to send any wounded to Pen Jewin, so if the war continues the way it has been we'll need wards to hold at least forty beds."

"How long do you think the war will last?" he asked me soulfully.

"Who can say? But we have to prepare for the worst if this whole area is to be taken care of. This is the only hospital servicing the areas of Kirkuk and Sul. Besides the Pesh Merga, there are many thousands of villagers depending on us." I paused to take a sip of tea, contemplating the vastness of the problem. Forty beds wasn't much to deal with so many people, but most of them could effectively be treated as out patients. Even so, if we were cut off and things became worse... "We have to build something big this time," I said firmly. "Big and permanent."

"Permanent?" Diman queried, looking at me as though I might have lost my tenuous grip on reality.

"Yes, permanent," I confirmed. "I want to build something for these people that will last."

Diman looked down into his empty teacup. I wondered if he might be looking for an inspirational solution in the remnants of his tealeaves as a gypsy fortuneteller might have done.

"I think I know where we can build," I added quietly.

Diman looked back up, searching my eyes for the answer.

"Near the cemetery," I explained. "Most of the area is well hidden."

"That's true, and there's plenty of water nearby..."

"And it's only three hundred meters from the village."

Diman stood up, seemingly energized. "When do we start?"

It was a big job, but with such dedicated and determined people by my side, nothing was impossible. I knew we'd have to start work immediately, and worry about getting financial support from the 4th section after it was too late for them to complain. Luckily there was no shortage of the raw materials we needed: mud, water, stones and

151

wood. All we needed was manpower, and for that we needed help from the local Party official. There was no shortage of labor either; it was more a matter of negotiating wages. Eventually we settled on half a pound for the workers, one pound for the bricklayer who would also function as an engineer, and one pound for those who brought donkeys with them. We never took anything from the villagers without compensating them; to do so was unthinkable in their circumstances. We paid for the mules we took on various missions, we paid for the wood to keep us warm, and we even paid for the vital work of transporting wounded, weapons and ammunition.

With the help of the Party official plans began to shape for the new hospital. There would be two separate wards, one for the men, and one a distance away for the women. In addition there would be a main facility building. Everything would be dug deep into the hillside so as three walls were completely buried, leaving only one side exposed for windows and doors, and that side would be hidden by trees. The roof would also be exposed, but likewise this would be easily disguised with mud and tree branches. Qualified engineers were a luxury we didn't have; it was only through experience, inspiration and a lot of luck that we would successfully be able to design and construct what would be the biggest thing ever built in this area. We took on twelve men to do the job, six for the main facility and three each for the two wards. To divert any flood waters a canal was excavated under the building. If memory serves we weren't two days into the job when we hit our first obstacle – literally. A gigantic rock was imbedded right where our quarry was taking place.

"We'll need the Brigade's bulldozer to move that," one of the workers told me.

"Why don't we just use dynamite?" another suggested.

I was against both ideas. The bulldozer was unreliable, and in any event I had not yet received permission from headquarters to be building this hospital. The dynamite might have worked, but it would have attracted some very unwelcome attention, so that didn't appear to be a valid option either. As I mused and mulled over the issue, one of the villagers piped up.

"I can move it," he said quietly.

I looked at him curiously.

152

"With the right men, I believe it can be done manually," he assured me.

I studied the rock, glanced back at the man, and was far less than convinced, but it was certainly worth a shot. I told him to hire the best people he could find, and he had my blessings to attempt this strenuous task. Within four weeks he'd accomplished what I would have considered impossible, while construction on the other buildings continued unimpeded. Over those four weeks a little mountain took shape comprised from pieces of chipped off rock – it was the sort of work that chain gangs in prison were forced to undertake as hard labor punishment, and these people did it willingly.

The next quandary we had to deal with was procuring furniture, sheets, windows, doors, and plenty of straw. Single-mindedly focused on the matter at hand, a group of our people set off to a deserted village on the far side of Daban where there were many abandoned public buildings. Although most had been damaged by bomb blasts, it was possible there would be a sufficient quantity of windows and doors to at least meet our needs. These committed individuals had to ferret around under the cover of darkness without a flashlight, without even smoking for fear the end of a lighted cigarette would alert the army to their presence. The journey was hazardous despite these precautions as both the Susei and Kanimeran garrisons often shelled the area just on the off-chance they might strike it lucky and hit some poor soul who was desperate enough to go scavenging among the ruins. It took several nights of meticulous foraging but the men eventually returned in relay with mules laden down by treasures; well, to us they were treasures. With a few nights work they found steel beds, steel doors, and steel window frames – a veritable treasure trove of goodies indeed.

With the winter hospital taking shape, I returned my attention full time to the patients who had need for my services in the summer hospital. One of the delightful little creatures who shared our land had become the most recent cause of a new and consistent problem. Leeches were finding their way into the water supply. Unsuspecting villagers taking a gulp of cool refreshing liquid in the dark were often the recipient of a very unwanted visitor to their gullets. No effective method for removing them had been developed; invariably we had to give the patient a specially designed solution to gargle with and when good fortune favored us, the offensive creatures would surface sufficiently for us to remove them with medical tweezers. It seemed there was no end to the creative methods by which a person could cause nauseating harm to oneself in the wilds of outback Kurdistan!

I visited the developing site of my new facility every day, supremely proud of the quick and efficient way it was progressing. All I needed to do now was get it paid for. The total cost of labor, materials and furniture had reached around three thousand Iraqi pounds. I couldn't put it off any longer. I had to take a deep breath and travel to Pen Jewin with a map of our new complex – and a bill for the work. Diman and I left by land-rover planning to pass the military outposts on the Asmar mountains after dark. It was a long and tiring trip, but it sure beat walking for a change.

I found it strangely comforting to see the village of Pen Jewin was as bustling as ever. The streets, cafés and restaurants were all full of people conducting trade in just about everything imaginable. It seemed since the fall of Sul that Pen Jewin had become the de facto business center for Iraqi Kurdistan. I didn't notice one face with the expression of distorted fear and fatigue that had become so familiar to me. It was almost as though the people here weren't at war at all. Quite remarkable.

After a quick breakfast we drove to the well-hidden hospital on the border of town in a small forest. This wasn't our final destination, but we needed to get permission to travel to the larger hospital of the 4th section from personnel on this side of the border, for across the other side of the border was Iran. The chief surgeon of our Movement was actually based in the Iranian city of Miriwan, where he was supplied with food, medicines and beds by the Iranian Red Cross. This was where all the most serious cases were treated – when they made it that far. Permission granted – we were on our way.

An eerie apprehension swept through me as Diman and I approached the military check point into Iran.

"We belong to the medical corps," I told them.

Once I was able to prove the validity of my claim our passage was approved, and within thirty minutes we were in the center of downtown Miriwan. It was a remarkably well-organized city with excellent shops, no shortage of restaurants and cafés, a sparkling public bath, and even a newly-erected movie theater. Although it was a Kurdish city, it was guarded by the mighty force of an Iranian army garrison. Everywhere I looked the place was swarming with Iranian soldiers – Iranian, but still Kurds. Even their accent was the same as the Kurds in Iraq. The more business-minded men from Sul had successfully secured management positions for themselves among the many thriving ventures in this area, and refugee camps housing around twelve thousand Kurds were only a few kilometers away, making it easy for our people to visit with their loved ones.

Again I couldn't help but be struck by the surreal contrasts that presented themselves in this nightmarish situation. On the one side thousands of people were being killed and injured on the front lines in Iraqi Kurdistan, yet here thousands more Kurds, both Pesh Merga and civilians, could enjoy a peaceful vacation. The concept was bizarre when the reality was we were in the middle of a war defending our very right to exist. I was probably still shaking my head with disbelief when I met with the chief surgeon from the hospital.

Not having visited this facility before it was with great pleasure that I accepted an invitation to tour the wards and see some of the patients I had patched up and sent across the border for further treatment. News of our achievements in Azad had spread widely, earning us great respect from all who met us. Even the local hotel owner, who was afraid to show his admiration openly for fear of the secret service who were known to infiltrate every nook and cranny of Kurdish occupied areas, quietly let us know how proud he was of our efforts. The chief surgeon, who understood our needs only too well, suggested we discuss the matter of finance in a civilized fashion over lunch. Lunch – the very idea of it set my saliva glands dancing. A proper meal, in a proper home, in a peaceful city – what an absolute luxury that would be!

After checking into our hotel I took a good look around the city. This was an entirely different world. It was as though no one here knew there was even a war being fought just miles away. The public bath was a sheer delight, large and clean with individual bathrooms that were well-heated and thoroughly comfortable. Well, perhaps 'thoroughly' comfortable was a bit of an overstatement – I did find it rather odd that the baths admitted men, children, *and* women! Everyone purchased their ticket and waited in line, and in between each customer the individual bathrooms were cleaned for the next patron. Truly it felt as though I'd just stepped into the 'Twilight Zone'!

Over lunch the entirely sympathetic chief surgeon took great pains to explain that although the building of winter hospitals had been approved, and he could plainly see our urgent need, the fact of the matter was that he had not yet received extra funds to assist. All he could offer us was four hundred pounds.

"But this won't come close to fulfilling our requirements," I complained. "Our oil lamps are old and weak. We have no sheets. There aren't enough blankets. I can't go back empty-handed."

"I understand," he said compassionately. "But my hands are tied. I can't give you that which I do not have."

"Perhaps then," I began slowly, rubbing my chin thoughtfully. "Perhaps you will permit me to travel to the main office in Noperdan, to make my plea directly."

"I will not only grant you such passage, but I'll write a letter of recommendation for you myself."

"Thank you," I sighed gratefully.

The following morning Diman and I headed off with the financial officer from the 4th section in an unlicensed land-rover. Since the war had begun there were no valid license plates for cars in the freed areas. Consequently we borrowed a number plate from one of the 4th section cars. Traveling in such relative comfort and security I must confess I was unable to resist a little self-indulgence. We were close to the Iranian city of Mahabad, which was once the capital of the Kurdish Republic. It wasn't exactly en route to Hajji Umran, which was our next destined stop, but it was a sight I had always wanted to see.

In 1964 Mahabad was declared a Kurdish Republic by Qazi Muhammed, a prominent politician of the time. The area included most of Iranian Kurdistan, and was dependent on Russia for developing its own army to protect themselves against the Iranian government, who back then was backed by the British and

Americans. While the Kurds apparently prospered under this administration, their fate was in fact being decided in Yalta. After only eleven months Qazi Muhammed and many of his ministers were arrested and hanged in the city square. In 1974, when I visited, the square was called Reza Pahlevi Square. A dot in the distance gradually grew in my vision until I found myself marveling at a huge statue of the Shah in the center of this square, proudly flanked by magnificent carvings of the king of all jungle beasts – the lion. It disgusted me to think that this too had been the scene of yet another brutal slaughter. But what appalled me more was the fact that the same injustice and oppression thrived to this very day.

As we crossed the border into Hajji Umran I saw thousands of refugees waiting for their papers. Suddenly the war was real again. Thousands of sad faces gazed on in hopeless wonder as we passed by. Thousands without homes. Thousands without shelter. If winter came early I couldn't comprehend the magnitude of the tragedy that would befall these people. The town itself was overflowing, and crawling with Pesh Merga. The overall picture was of a war that wasn't going to end any time soon. The cars were all covered in mud, or painted gray/green. The road was virtually lined with anti-aircraft batteries. And everywhere we went all the talk was about the war.

Our armaments were woefully inferior to the opposing forces. Rumors were rife that soon we would be rewarded for our sacrifices with more modern and effective weapons, however seeing the rumors materialize into something more tangible was apparently a special kind of magic I was unlikely to witness. This brutal war had been raging for fourteen years with only minor hiccups. With the first casualty of war being the truth, it was perhaps inevitable that rumors without substance would be endemic. I dare say some even had us believing that the Shah was really helping the Movement, by way of justifying what was in fact a total sellout to his regime. However these rumors did serve a positive purpose. Somehow they helped us believe that against impossible odds, even though we were outnumbered and outgunned, we could still win victory in a glorious triumph of the faithful and the proud. While belief held strong that miraculous marvelous weapons would one day magically appear, our ability to continue the fight with an outdated arsenal never waned.

Of course the Ba'ath regime was no stranger to spreading rumors either. One of their more creative efforts was an attempt to convince their army that the Movement was comprised only of a small clique serving the interests of imperialistic powers. This fascist fairytale served to create an illusion that Iraq was really at war with Iran, which could at least go part way to explaining their heavy losses and help justify why they went after the oil rich fields of Kirkuk.

When Diman and I returned from our trip to Panjuwin I went with the dresser on duty to attend to people who had come from a village about a half hour away. One of the Pesh Merga I knew well needed my help with his wife who had been in labor for the last three days without being able to deliver her baby. She was in a very serious condition. In fact the midwife had told the Pesh Merga that if his wife didn't receive help soon she would likely die. I was advised the family wanted a nurse in attendance and the woman's father, a Hagie (a man who had been to Mecca), gave his greetings and urged the nurse to come at once.

There was little I could do about their decision-making process. Usually the men frowned on their wives or next of kin being examined by a man, but until recently there had been no other option. Now that we had an experienced nurse and midwife most people wanted her to attend the sick women. As the father was a Hagie the situation was even more difficult. I decided it best to concede to their wishes as it was better for the woman to have help from a midwife than no help at all. I sent for Laila, explained the situation to her, and asked her to go. I told the Diman to assist and if necessary induce birth, instructing him to take an infusion and other appropriate medicines with him. It must have been around midnight when they left, disappearing into the darkness, walking somberly on a black and moonless night. Happily, around ten the next morning, Diman and Lila returned after completing a successful mission.

CHAPTER TWELVE

Within an hour of meeting with the health headquarters in Noperdan I received all the financial assistance I'd requested. They also approved in advance an allocation for our food supplies from November until March the following year, which was an enormous boost to our efforts. Thanks to their generosity and foresight we would be able to secure all the supplies we were going to need before the winter season set in and we were cut off from any external supply routes. With three and a half thousand pounds in our pocket, Diman and I hurried to the city of Kirmenshah in Iran, where we spent the following two days buying up everything we could get our hands on. By the time we returned to Pen Jewin all we needed was food. After a few pleasantries, and several cups of tea, we commenced our jubilant return to Azad in a convoy of one land-rover, two trucks, and a tractor with a fully loaded trailer.

Tears filled my eyes on seeing my beautiful and beloved Azad once again materialize before me. It would be impossible to describe how much I loved this place, and given the horrendous circumstances I dare say for most it would be impossible to understand why. But such is the physical natural beauty of this mountainous region, such is the purity of heart of its people, and so valiant is their determination to survive, I truly could have lived a thousand years there with no desire to experience the richness of the rest of the world. Too many times during our return journey it seemed as though I would never see this place again. Traveling under cover of darkness without headlights was not only tedious but also dangerous, and even then the noise of our tractor made us easily detectable to nearby troops. We were shot at and bombed several times as we rolled ever closer to our precious

Azad, yet all the might the enemy threw at us happily amounted to naught.

During our absence the women's ward had been successfully completed. It was as though we could almost breathe again. We had enough money, medicines and food to last us six months – it was a cause for celebration – and a very timely one with the feast of Ramadan upon us.

The construction of the main hospital building hadn't been quite as successful as the women's ward. Our old friend, the giant rocks, had once again played a part in impeding progress. We had two weeks to clear the area in order to start building and have the brickwork dry before forced relocation would commence. Two weeks to achieve what quite reasonably should have taken several months. However, the rest of the complex was looking good. From the women's ward I strolled along a small rock path through grapevines and luscious trees to the men's ward. Everything was coming together nicely. The main surgical ward was also complete, with capacity for sixteen beds, a small dressing room and a separate section for the dresser on duty. The building quite literally looked as though it was smiling at me as the sunlight glinted off its newly fitted steel-framed windows and doors. On another nearby hillside the isolation ward was almost ready. This was a vital component for the hospital as we received so many cases of tuberculosis, viral hepatitis, meningitis, and typhoid fever.

The men were paid in full for their labors as soon as I returned home. We also paid for over three hundred trees that had been used to construct our new ceilings. All in all, we were in pretty good shape, so much so in fact that I discussed with Diman the possibility of constructing an out-patient building with the several tons of broken rock that were now idly piled into a newly created mini mountain. I also wanted to explore the possibility of building a water pipeline. Although there was a water supply nearby, it was arduous work for both man and beast to continually carry sufficient quantities for our needs. With barley being as expensive as bread, the donkey that was destined to servitude was not always fed as much as he should have been. The poor thing would escape at every opportunity to run off and find a fresh food supply. On top of that, two people had to work fourteen-hour days every day, to fill the water and walk to and fro with our overworked and underfed beast of burden.

Diman came up with the notion that we could build a pipeline from a spring near where his parents lived, three kilometers away. It was separated from the village by many hills and valleys, but this actually turned out to be an ironic advantage. Steel piping was far too expensive for our meager budget; instead we purchased six thousand meters of three quarter inch plastic tubing in five hundred meter lengths, which cost us seventy precious pounds. It was a big gamble because if the spring turned out not to be high enough to create the necessary pressure to pump the water through we'd have burned a relatively large percentage of our allowance. But this is where the hills and valleys came into their own. As the water reached the top of a hill the slope produced sufficient acceleration to force the water across to the next hill. Of course our ingenious pipeline had to be well buried otherwise it would freeze up during the winter months. If any of the sections of piping became loose or damaged once buried we'd be sunk, for it would have been impossible to locate where the problem was within three kilometers of ground covered by several feet of snow.

If our crazy plan worked, Diman and I decided we'd sell the donkey for twenty pounds to save him from the murderous work he was forced to undertake. We'd save ten pounds a month in costs for his barley, plus the expense of paying two people to labor gruelingly alongside him. Piece by piece we began tying the five hundred meter sections together, and placed a filter at one end to sieve out dirt and other unwanted contaminants, such as the grotesque leeches. We allowed our conduit to function for several days before we were confident this patchwork masterpiece wouldn't fall apart, at which time it was securely buried underground.

Meanwhile, the never-ending stream of sick and injured continued to flood in. I have to admit at times I not only felt exhaustion beyond any measure I could comprehend, but I could see that stress and despondency were mounting like an insidious cancer. People were operating on a short fuse. The slightest dispute could escalate into World War III within a heartbeat, forcing me to grant more vacation time than I would have liked. Political unrest was also on the rise. For the first time it was apparent that the people were starting to mistrust the methods of their leadership. This wasn't helped by hearing broadcasts by the Movement on the radio asserting our losses were less serious than we knew them to me – we knew because we were personally knitting pieces of Pesh Merga back together again. Lies and propaganda didn't hold water when the blood of your brethren trickled unerringly through your hands.

Rumors, rumors, and more rumors. Rumors about impending negotiations with the fascist government. Rumors that the Movement was going to receive heavy modern weapons. Rumors that the leadership was going to declare a one-sided autonomous government. Rumors that the refugees in Iran were going to receive more money, better houses and camps to live in. Rumors that something big was going to happen any day. No one could distinguish fact from fantasy any longer, yet despite this heavy burden we continued to successfully treat patients in the summer hospital as the winter hospital neared total completion. Every family in Azad volunteered at least one member of their household to help us out for two days a week free of charge. Those who had no men in their households brought mule loads of wood for the winter. Before winter set in we had enough wood to last us through the season, something we never would have dreamed possible.

Once the water pipeline was functional for the hospital, I began exploring the possibility of improving the water supply for the village at large. Up until this point the pure, clean spring water that serviced the village was used not only for drinking but also for washing needs. This included people, clothes, and animals. In addition, the water supply attracted the many insects of the area like moths to a flame, including of course the malaria carrying mosquitoes. I wanted to build a cement enclosure around the spring with numerous taps that could facilitate a higher level of sanitation. With a little extra effort I considered it would also be possible to extend the pipeline through the two main sections of the village, putting taps at fifty meter intervals. If I could achieve this people living as far away as two or three kilometers from the spring wouldn't have to make the long journey several times a day to collect water. This task was always carried out by women and girls, most of whom were no older than nine years. It was heavy work that created many back deformities as a result.

The spring water supply was on a hill, which was a good start. We still had plenty of raw materials to build with, what we needed was cement. I drafted an official letter to the health department in one of the border towns in Iran, requesting one thousand pounds of the concrete necessary to carry out the job. As I understand it, my letter was never even read. This situation presented yet another of the cruel ironic contradictions of this land. One of the most precious gifts of life, water, was in abundance, yet it was also the major source of illness. People drinking contaminated water often suffered infections, including tuberculosis. Those who swallowed leeches suffered internal bleeding and anemia. These sinister little black monsters were often tiny when they entered a person's throat, but by gorging themselves on blood, they grew quickly until they were nestled in a swamp of coagulated blood that caused ulceration. When these insidious vampires couldn't be removed from the throat with medical tweezers we had to get very creative with our treatment. Sometimes a sedative would induce them to return to the surface, other times a concentration of citric juices or salt water would do the trick. But in some cases the patients didn't come to see me until they were already well in shock and requiring an infusion. One particular victim required blood transfusions as it took a full fourteen days before we could convince the determined and vile creature to pop out.

By the end of September the temperature was already beginning to drop. The wind was wild in the wilderness, and the rains had started to fall early. Happily the winter hospital was just about ready. In early October the patients were moved into the facility, and I gave ten days leave to everyone who had labored so tirelessly to achieve this impossible dream. In truth I must confess I granted the leave partly out of gratitude and compassion, and partly because the peoples' poor hands were so raw and blistered they wouldn't have been able to work anyway. For the first time in ten months I felt I could rest easy, and in the blissful isolation of privacy. Oh for just a little peace and quiet – but it was not to be ...

163

I had no sooner settled in for a quiet night when the village was hit by a heavy round of artillery from the Susei garrison. It was as though they knew where my hospital was. Miraculously no damage was done, but I was certain the target of the shelling was no coincidence. They had never bombed that area of the village before, and while they did miss the hospital the explosions were in precariously close proximity. Perhaps it *was* just coincidence? I chose to try and convince myself of that fact, hearing heavenly silence once more descend upon my world. Ah, finally, a little peace and quiet. I would dearly have loved to read a novel, but that would have been a ridiculously extravagant luxury. There were no novels to read. Instead I recreated one I remembered in my mind, 'Crime and Punishment'. Somehow it seemed appropriate. I was just beginning to doze off when I heard strange voices outside. Snapping into full alert I reached for my Klashnikov, cocked it and set it on automatic.

"Who's there?" I demanded, once I was safely ensconced behind the relative safety of my Russian automatic weapon.

"Brother doctor, we have brought you a sick Pesh Merga."

"Of course," I mumbled under my breath, putting my gun aside and heading to the front door.

Blinking through the darkness I could make out four Pesh Merga holding a fifth. The gentle silvery gaze of a full moon washed over him. For once it was plain to see that the condition was not too serious, however the flickering moonlight behind him reminded me of another late night emergency I'd been called to only a few weeks earlier …

"Brother doctor, come quickly," I was summoned by a night guard. "There's a young boy, he's badly wounded and waiting in the dressing room."

I rushed towards the scene of the commotion to find an eleven-year-old child wrapped in a blanket. Ahmed held an oil lamp near the boy for me to inspect the situation. He was pale and motionless, perhaps already dead. His cold arm was pulseless and his blood pressure unreadable. Quickly I instructed Ahmed to raise the rear legs of the table while I prepared an infusion. The boy's upper arm was virtually amputated, and the bone smashed to smithereens. Every important blood vessel and nerve seemed to be destroyed, and there was massive blood loss. As usual everyone on hand was prepared to donate blood, but on this occasion I was the only one whose type matched. The dresser on duty was the least experienced in taking blood, and I knew if he inadvertently pushed an air bubble into my veins while siphoning, well it would have been curtains for brother doctor – and his patient. Fortunately I was siphoned without incident.

I had to complete the amputation very high up on the boy's arm to find enough skin to cover the stump. With my blood and strong sedatives pumping through his veins, the process began. As I operated on the child I found myself once again wondering if I might be losing my mind as I could hear singing! The soft angelic tones of a child singing! Looking towards the boy's sweet, young face I discovered the source of this strange melody – it was the child himself! His voice was so weak I could hardly make out the words over the sound of his father's sobbing grief. Although his father was outside the melancholy music had drifted towards him, clearly opening a still fresh wound in his aching heart. It was a bizarre and bittersweet episode in our own never-ending series of 'beauty and the beast' – the beauty of love and hope, the beast of war and suffering.

It took another two hours to complete the operation, but within two weeks the child was strong enough to be discharged. The 4th section had promised us that all amputees would receive artificial limbs; a promise I conveyed to the boy in good faith. At fortnightly intervals he would visit me, amazingly upbeat, but always with the same question.

"Has my new arm arrived from Iran yet?"

"Not yet," I told him, trying to sound cheerful. "But any day now, I'm sure."

"There's no hurry," the boy cheered. "The school isn't starting this year anyway."

"I see," I replied, choking back the tears I wanted to shed. "And what is it you want to do when you grow up?"

"I did want to be a Pesh Merga, like my father. But now father says I should become a teacher." For the first time the confidence in his little voice broke as his gaze trailed towards the stump on his right shoulder. "But I don't know if I can write with my left arm," he almost whimpered in a whispering tone.

"Of course you can," I boomed. "Look, I can write with my left hand." I quickly gave him a demonstration, which he seemed to find quite fascinating.

Over time I grew quite close to the boy on his regular fortnightly visits, but with a heavy heart I have to admit I never did live to see him receive his new arm.

∞∞

Ominous clouds heralded the impending arrival of winter as I quietly thanked whatever powers there were that we were prepared to take on whatever the fates chose to throw at us. For the first time I even had a real headquarters, a home that had been deserted with four rooms, including one I was able to keep all to myself. There was even a well-maintained bathroom. Luxury! The house was built in a valley with the roof at earth level on three sides, disguising us from aerial attacks. The sole drawback was the chimney. Government agents had taken to throwing grenades down chimneys just as a household gathered around the fire to warm themselves for the evening. I resolutely determined the army would receive no joy if they tried that little maneuver on us. Diman and I collected a bunch of long nails and hammered them across the chimney flue so close together that a grape couldn't squeeze through.

The arrival of winter was every inch as bitter as we'd anticipated, although the snow-covered roads that led to our village did nothing to slow down the continuous flood of sick and wounded to our doors. It wasn't until well into November, when heavy snow covered the high mountains, that the stream of people began diminishing to a trickle. My mornings started routinely with two cups of tea and five cigarettes before heading to the hospital. Day after long and disheartening day the monotonous ritual was unrelenting. Night after night I'd trudge home, light my fire, and gaze into the flames of pure hell wondering if there would ever be any respite. During those winter months I was too often alone with my thoughts as I lost myself in the timeless images of the blaze before me. I began to doubt. It was just a seed of doubt at first, but each night it seemed to sprout a new

166

root, a new leaf, a new branch until it was almost overpowering me. I suddenly realized I was working for a leadership whose policy I no longer believed in. Although, I was working for the people I loved, to try and save their lives, what was it all for if there was no happy conclusion to this state of affairs? Was I finally beginning to lose my fragile grip on sanity?

∞∞

The winter was well entrenched when I received an urgent message to head to Sargelow. The Brigade's commander was suffering from chronic kidney damage and had been transported to the hospital in Pen Jewin. This left a former army lieutenant in his place, although it was obvious to anyone that the commander had already been delegating any real responsibility to the younger man who was a former army officer. Fate can indeed be a strange thing for the younger officer was Kurdo, the Kurd who'd deserted from the Iraqi army and I'd met when I was first assigned to the general hospital in Sul. It was a warm and welcome reuniting of kindred spirits. When I left Sul I didn't think I'd ever see Kurdo again, and now here he was taking charge of a Brigade for the Movement and in more ways than one a Godsend for me.

My dear friend Kurdo refused to let me leave Sargelow without first giving me a small electric generator, sixteen gallons of gasoline to run it with, forty 60 volt bulbs, some conducting wire, and a healthy mule to carry it all. These items were of immeasurable value for the frequent nighttime operations we'd previously had to conduct by the light of nothing more than an oil lamp. I'd long ago been promised a generator for my hospital, but as was increasingly common this was a promise that was never honored. Once Kurdo was in de facto command I quickly became the proud parent of my very own little generator. He even sent a Pesh Merga who was qualified as an electro-technician to help us set up the necessary circuits to bring electricity to my hospital. I don't think I had ever been so pleased to see anyone in all my life.

The villagers' eyes sparkled like children witnessing their first Christmas tree lights when the marvel of electricity was established in Azad. Even though the electricity was only for the hospital, it was nevertheless considered a momentous occasion. Increasingly it was annoying me that these people could be so easily impressed by utilities that most of the world's population took for granted. More and more I yearned to be with the Pesh Merga where the real action was, instead of patching up the damage afterwards. A deep loathing was beginning to fester in my heart and soul; it was a screaming restless silence that couldn't be subdued.

I had received an invitation to cross the great mountain of Pira Magron to visit my dear friend, Kurdo, on the other side. He'd been injured twice during the past seven months, and while he'd been recuperating in my facility our friendship had grown stronger than ever. Kurdo was one of the bravest and most noble men I knew, and he was right in the thick of the main action. In a way I envied him. I considered myself a revolutionary and wanted to be in the thick of the action too. Whether it was morally or medically, I wanted to be all I could be, give all I could give. And I wanted to take Kurdo up on his invitation. The plan was for us to meet Kurdo at the Headquarters of the 6th Battalion in a small village near Sul between the high ragged mountains of Daban and Pira Magron. Emerging from the bosom of Mother Nature's giants a joint action of 3rd and 6th battalions was to take place against an army garrison in Sul. Afterwards, with God's help, we were to cross the big Pira Magron to reach the 3rd Battalion on the other side led by Anwar.

While contemplating the wisdom of this trip over dinner one night, a villager commented to me, "Our war is like the train trip from Baghdad to Basra. The train stops at stations en route, people get off and others get on, but regardless the train moves on to reach its final destination."

It was an intriguing analogy, and true in so far as many who start a revolution do not remain alive to see it through to its conclusion. But a revolution needs more than one driving force – its generals – for with only one train, if it derails the end destination will never be reached. The entire ugly unholy debacle of this war had my senses reeling. Yet even as I seriously considered crossing the great Pira

Magron mountain my services were called upon to provide another gruesome duty.

Thirty high school students had been sequestered to join the newly formed chemical warfare department. Among the many rampant rumors circulating in Iraq, one which seemed to have taken hold was that the government would soon be using poison gas to break the spirit of our revolution. The students had been tasked with traveling from village to village to train people how to protect themselves from such an event. It was a ludicrous exercise in futility as there weren't more than eight hundred gas masks in the whole of Iraqi Kurdistan, and not a single shelter capable of protecting more than a hundred people. If the government did use this most dreaded of weapons, the affected area could reach over one million people and the Kurds didn't possess more than a few kilos of chemicals capable of neutralizing the poison. Once again, despite preposterously impossible odds, these people would not be intimidated, and so it fell to me to train the young students how to care for the injured and administer injections. Why? Why, why, why, why, why, why, why, why, why?

If there was any silver lining to this cloud perhaps it was that the students eventually became skilled dressers. A few of them in fact became Pesh Merga themselves; a situation that sadly led to an unpleasant demise for too many who bravely marched on down that path. But horror does breed heroes, and sometimes they come from the most unlikely quarters. While I never considered myself a hero, the fact was I didn't have to remain in Kurdistan, or even Iraq. I had chosen to be there. However, I was Iraqi. I was born and raised in Iraq and although I wasn't a Kurd, indeed I wasn't even Muslim, I did think of these people as my own. In other words I felt I had a duty because I felt a kinship. The same could surely not be said for a young French doctor who volunteered to work in several front line hospitals direct from graduating medical school. Time and again this man put his life on the line, crisscrossing the country, speaking with high officials, and keeping extensive notes on everything he encountered. I had the good fortune to work with him for several weeks when his expedition brought him into Azad, and consequently led to another adventure.

It was late in December when I finally accepted the invitation to cross the Pira Magron mountain, but this was no social call. I'd received a telegram stating the 3rd battalion was badly in need of expert medical assistance, so without hesitation I readied the best dresser we had, the healthiest mule in the village, and its owner. I assigned Diman to take care of my hospital with our young French visitor, thinking it was fortuitous timing indeed for a guest appearance by a fellow physician. So much for what I thought ...

"You can't be serious," I gasped.

"I am very serious," the French doctor assured me in a deeply solemn voice.

"But if you are caught by the enemy you will be shot on the spot as a spy, because you're ..."

"French?"

"Foreign."

"I have not come to Iraq to sit back safely while people can benefit from my care."

I looked around the area, wondering what his concept of 'safely' was exactly.

"I can manage, brother doctor," Diman assured me.

I just shook my head. I certainly could use the extra pair of hands, but even taking into account the time this French doctor had already spent in Iraq I doubted he had any concept of what trials lay in store.

The mule owner who traveled with us was a great storyteller. At times this lightened our mood, while on other occasions it was a distinct curse. He knew the area well, a little too well in terms of expounding some of the potential horrors that could await us. In translating each story for the Frenchman I was continually amazed at his ability to remain calm. If he was unnerved by any of this, he certainly wasn't showing it. He learned how to catch a live rabbit in the snow: by following paw prints that would lead to a snow-covered lair, visible only by the rising warm mist of the rabbit's breathing from inside. En route, in Sargelow, he learned that the government's economic blockade had little effect on a people living in a land so rich in natural resources. In truth the Kurdish people could have been entirely self-sufficient with good-planning and good-management, but the Movement didn't even try to become self-sufficient.

In my increasingly disillusioned state I was beginning to see with a crystallizing clarity that rhetoric was equally as destructive from one warring faction as it was from another. The Movement argued that the Kurdish people were one class, and to attempt self-sufficiency would mean dividing their people into classes. Their slogan was, *One people, One Class, One Cause.* What nonsense! The reality of the matter was that five percent of the people were brutal landlords who controlled all the fertile land and treated the long-suffering peasants as part of their livestock. As that thought tumbled through my mind I wondered if I'd became jaded, or whether this was realism? Perhaps it was a little of both.

CHAPTER THIRTEEN

I really can't recall what led to a plan to march headlong into the front lines. Perhaps it was the young French doctor's insistence on being part of a military mission, I honestly don't remember with the passage of time. It seems strange now that I'm calling the French doctor 'young'. Physically I wasn't that much older than the Frenchman, yet I felt a century his senior. My eyes had seen too much. Certainly I had no lust or curiosity to witness a battle firsthand, but then I had to remind myself I'd already enjoyed that so-called privilege on too many occasions. Whatever prompted it, the Pesh Merga guiding us decided there was a simple mission we could carry out and suddenly we were each handed two bazooka rockets to carry. I stuck one in each pocket of my overcoat, thinking they didn't weigh too much even though I was already carrying my Kalashnikov and a pistol.

In my dreams I think I will forever be trudging up treacherously jagged paths on frozen mountain ranges. If the way to get to know a land is on foot, then truly I shall never know any land as intimately as I came to know Iraqi Kurdistan. Quickly I lost count of the number of times I fell before we reached a tiny hut, the last Pesh Merga outpost before our chosen passage. Our Pesh Merga guides proudly told the Pesh Merga of the area what their military objective was.

"It won't work," one of the locals said simply.

"Why not?" our Pesh Merga asked.

"Because the fog is so thick the soldiers will be inactive."

"Then we'll wait until sunrise."

"If it's like the last few days, the fog won't lift until late in the morning."

172

"Well, we'll just see what it's like in the morning," our Pesh Merga huffed.

Come morning, the prediction proved accurate. We could hardly see our hands in front of our faces, although on scanning our motley crew it was plain enough to see that none of those faces looked happy.

"As I told you," the local said wisely. "To carry out the mission you have in mind would mean waiting until late in the day, and by then the tanks from the Susei garrison will be on the highway with guns pointed at your passage. You won't stand a chance."

I quietly breathed a heavy sigh of relief, hoping my traveling companions didn't notice the huge billowing mist that escaped from my lips into the freezing air. I was a doctor. I was trained to save lives, not take them. Okay, I carried a gun to protect myself, and I did have a burning desire to travel with the Pesh Merga on their missions, but not for the purpose of taking life. All I wanted was to be on hand when they needed me most, and I'm certain my French colleague felt the same. However, to a soldier, guerilla, or other trained slayer, life had become a continuous session of kill or be killed. I guess, given that choice, I know which side of the fence I would want to be sitting on. I hadn't thought the plan our Pesh Merga guides had come up with was that 'sporting' in the first place. Although I guess that was the whole point – the more certain the enemy's death, and the more certain your survival, the better the plan. But at the end of the day many of the army's soldiers were just kids who'd been taken forcibly from their families to fight a battle they didn't believe in and didn't understand. It was all an enigma wrapped in a puzzle tied up in a riddle – IT WAS ALL MADNESS!

They kill, we kill, and they kill back. Where does it end? When there's no one left to murder or brutalize any longer? And for what? A difference in the way we tie our shoelaces or prayed to the same one Almighty being? IT WAS MADNESS!

Did God really care if you prayed standing up, sitting down, in a temple, or in the middle of grass field? How over-inflated is man's opinion of himself that he considers we matter enough to be of such significance? Or was the truth closer to the fact that all these wars, the wars of mankind throughout the ages, were rarely anything truly to do with religious beliefs at all? Perhaps the truth more closely lies with individual leaders' insatiable lust for power and control over an ever-increasing dominion, especially when that dominion was rich with a resource that could increase one's material wealth. MADNESS!

We withdrew. Praise whatever powers there were – we withdrew, crossing to the safe(r) side near the Pesh Merga checkpoint that led down to a village. From there we could continue unimpeded to the headquarters of the 6th battalion, led by my dear friend Kurdo.

No sooner had we left the village than it began to snow, reminding me of a story told around campfires for generations about a small village in this area. A family with seven sons lived in one of the modest dwellings, so the story goes. Their father was wise, and accustomed to the harsh climatic conditions of the region. When a heavy snow storm began that could have lasted for days or even weeks, the father immediately realized their situation posed a clear and present danger. In preparation for the arduous time ahead, the father sent his sons out to butcher all the livestock they possessed before they froze to death. With that accomplished, he built a fire and sent two sons at a time out to shovel snow away from the roof of the house until they became too weary to continue, at which point two other sons would take over. While the weary sons rested they were treated to a meal of roast meat.

According to the legend, which dates back hundreds of years, this routine continued for two weeks until the snow storm finally halted. At that point the family emerged to discover they were the only survivors in the village. The other homes remained covered in meters of snow until the following spring when their inhabitants were all found frozen to death in their crumbled abodes. Since then the area has been considered almost holy, a shrine to the will, endurance, and determination of the Kurdish people. I held onto that thought as I trudged through the ever worsening conditions, looking forward to a warm welcome, and even warmer cup of tea, when I finally reached Kurdo.

It was like arriving at an oasis in the desert when the 6th Battalion headquarters finally came into view.

"Kurdo," I gushed, on catching sight of my friend. "It's so good to see you."

"You too, brother doctor. There are many in urgent need of your care here."

I was, of course, only too happy to be able to offer aid and comfort to the ailing. However, after treating the sick and wounded for several hours my relative sense of self-worth was suddenly crushed. I listened in dismay as I learned I had escaped the frying pan only to leap headfirst directly into the fire. The 6th battalion, together with a group of Pesh Merga from Kurdo's 4th battalion, was planning an attack on Sul. Both my French colleague and I were invited to attend the party, but it was ultimately decided having a foreigner on hand was too great a risk. Instead we were to be given the privilege of taking up a position on a nearby hill with ringside seats for the battle ahead. After a hearty lunch we headed off on a three-hour trek towards our date with destiny. The Pesh Merga were armed with light automatic weapons, hand grenades in their belts, and two of them carried anti-tank guns.

It was hard to imagine that when I first met Kurdo he had been an army deserter. Who could have dreamt that he would become a Battalion commander and I would be a first-hand witness to his courageous acts of daring as he marched his men directly into the jaws of hell? I couldn't help but admire his strength, determination and unwavering dedication to his people. Before we parted company on this particular mission, Kurdo headed for battle and I to observe, I allowed myself to soak in some of his charismatic fortitude thinking what a privilege it was to know this man.

Our band of rebels was forty strong when we reached the final Pesh Merga checkpoint, where we collected a further one hundred troops. During this brief pit stop I could do nothing to treat the ailing children of the area – there was no time. With sad eyes and a heavy heart I studied their gloomy little faces. The only creature who truly looked healthy was a large white cat who caught two mice while I was watching him. Was this the universe's way of telling me that death and killing was simply a natural part of life?

With the battalion's complement complete, the Pesh Merga readied themselves for battle. It was, for want of a better word, an impressive sight to see that many men armed and in uniform with a single thought of purpose, yet all I could think about was how many of them would be coming back.

Outside the village two RBG 7s were tested. They functioned well. It was not unheard of for Pesh Merga to stand as close as fifty yards from a military convoy simply to test the functioning capacity of their enemy's firepower. The reward for such bravery was certain death. I'd once seen a Pesh Merga who'd volunteered for this duty with over a hundred machine-gunned bullet holes in his body. Another had managed to escape with his bowels in his hand. Incredibly he made it all the way to the nearest village, four kilometers away, before collapsing dead in his own entrails minutes later.

The Frenchman and I parted company with the main fighting force at the end of a symbolically shaky bridge. The foreigner, three Pesh Merga and myself went one way, while the rest of the battalion, led by Kurdo, marched forward into the fray. There was no time for goodbyes, no time for good luck wishes, just a clinical separation from the Pesh Merga who headed towards certain death and destruction (of one side or the other). Taking up our position behind large rocks I glanced down at a village below. A charming restaurant and café had been built around a small artificial lake. They were deserted now, of course. I couldn't help thinking how lonely they looked, isolated from their patrons who were their purpose for being. At this time of day they should have been bustling with the sound of cheerful chatter, the decibels rising over clinking glasses. But no, they were silent. The air was silent. Everything was deathly silent, until …

BOOM!

It had begun. The cement factory was hit first, the blast extinguishing lights as though someone had simply snuffed out a candle. It took only moments for the counter offensive to hit back from three separate directions. Even in our supposedly relatively safe position the mortar fire came perilously close. The elder Pesh Merga among us ordered my colleague and I to take cover – an order that didn't need to be given twice. For every round our side fired at the troops they must have fired thirty by return. It didn't take long for the battle to extend into Sul itself, with the sound of heavy machinegun fire and tanks moving in on the area. Car and street lights in the city were all switched off. It was dark – very dark. And it was cold – cold, dark – and terribly sad. I couldn't take it any more. I made the unilateral decision to head down the hill to the nearest village.

Good for the Pesh Merga. They had Sul under their control. Now I wanted to go inside somewhere it was warm, and if I was lucky I might even find a friendly face.

The nearest village was also in blackness. The only sound was my leaden footsteps. Not even the dogs were barking.

A local man invited me into his home. He was friendly enough, although he was plainly cogitating over the likelihood of his village being the next target once the fighting stopped in Sul. Thirty minutes later my French colleague and our Pesh Merga joined me. I looked upon my foreign colleague with a combination of pity and rebuke, noticing he had that look in his eyes – the look of a man who would never forget what he had just witnessed.

Before we had parted company at the shaky bridge, Kurdo had instructed us to rendezvous with the rest of the Pesh Merga battalion in the next village at midnight. Our escorts took us directly to a home where Kurdo would meet us, in the event he survived the battle that is. Time and again I wondered if this time would be the last time I would lay eyes on my dear friend. Anxiously I waited in silence as each second ticked noisily by. Each tick of the clock seemed to last an eternity as the dismal waiting continued and I had no option but to endure the agonizing uncertainty of the fate of my friend.

Just after midnight the first group of Pesh Merga arrived, carrying one of their brethren.

"Is he badly wounded?" I asked.

"No, brother doctor. He's frozen."

"Frozen?!"

"Yes. We had to walk through streams on our way to Sul."

"Bring him to the stove," I ordered.

He was soaked to the bone and shivering like the last autumn leaf on a denuded tree.

"My feet," he cried painfully.

The poor man was immediately given fresh clothes and wrapped in blankets.

"What of the others?" I asked no one in particular.

177

"We are all uninjured, but Serwan has been left behind."

"Serwan?" my eyebrows raised.

"What is it?" the French doctor asked, seeing my shock. I translated the conversation thus far.

"I remember Serwan," the Frenchman announced in mild shock. "We treated him for acute kidney infection not ten days ago."

"That's him," I confirmed.

"How could he be left behind? I remember you ordered him to take a month's sick leave. Besides, I don't remember seeing him with the rest of the Pesh Merga."

"That's a good point," I conceded, turning to the Pesh Merga and switching languages. "Serwan wasn't with you when we left, was he?"

"No. He joined us in the village, after we separated from you."

"But kaka Najmeden knew he was sick and supposed to be resting."

"That's true, but kaka doctor, Serwan insisted on coming. He said he would shoot himself if we didn't let him come."

"But he's only seventeen years old," I mumbled to myself.

Suddenly everyone fell silent. We all knew 'left behind' meant captured, and that didn't mean anything good.

A moment later twenty pale, quiet Pesh Merga joined us fresh from the battle, accompanied by Kurdo.

"What about Serwan?" I asked.

"He could still make it back," a thirty-year-old Pesh Merga said, trying hopelessly to sound positive. "Perhaps he got lost."

"Do you really believe that?" Kurdo growled.

"No, brother, I don't," the Pesh Merga replied in a husky voice of shame.

"Why didn't you do as I instructed?" Kurdo demanded.

"The plan didn't turn out the way we thought."

"Why? Wasn't the door open?"

"No."

"So why didn't you just blow it open?" Kurdo barked angrily. "You had machine guns and hand grenades."

178

"We did, but it took time. When we reached the second floor we could hear tanks rolling towards the building. We had to shoot our way out as it was."

"So why didn't you use the RBG against the tanks?"

"There were six of them! We had no chance."

"So what did you do?" Kurdo blustered.

"We joined Ali's group as planned."

Kurdo stiffened. "Where's Ali?"

"He'll be here soon."

"Bring him to me! And he'd better have a damned good explanation or by the grave of my brother I will have him executed this very night."

I later learned that the Pesh Merga who had entered the city were divided into several small groups, each with a certain task under a designated leader. The group leader who was being grilled before me was supposed to retrieve something from the building he'd had to fight his way into. The precise military tactics and their overall strategy were never discussed openly in front of civilians, as successful operations were often repeated. In any event, I had no interest in their tactics or strategy. All I cared about, and all the Pesh Merga cared about, was that it was shameful to leave a man behind. All their faces screamed with expressions of the deep pain they felt on losing a brother without actually knowing what had happened to him.

Another Pesh Merga arrived. He wasn't inside the door when Kurdo ripped into him. "What happened after you ran from …?"

"It wasn't what you think," the man interrupted him.

"Then tell me how it was!" Kurdo roared.

"The army had blocked all the main roads. We had to take side roads to reach Ali and the others. It took us almost forty minutes."

"Was Ali in his location?"

"We were about fifty meters away when suddenly heavy firing began in our direction. We were caught by surprise and couldn't fire back because Ali and the others were in the middle. The attack was aimed at Ali, not us, but he couldn't fire back because the assault was so heavy."

"Why didn't you use the RBG against the building?"

"I didn't know who was inside."

179

Kurdo pounded his fist, bellowing, "You saw fire coming from the building, didn't you?"

"Fire was coming from many directions."

Kurdo grimaced in silence for a few seconds.

"I crawled to Ali," the Pesh Merga continued quietly. "I asked him what was going on. He told me to go with my people and wait for them on the outskirts of the city. He didn't mention anything about Serwan being captured."

At that moment the man in question arrived. Tall, thin, tired and depressed, Ali trudged into our room still carrying his RBG. The area was dimly lit, and during the course of the debrief it had become thick with cigarette smoke. Nonetheless it was plain to see the gaze of these two men lock with fervor.

"Tell me the truth," Kurdo growled in a low rumbling voice.

Ali stared back at his commander, not afraid, not even disturbed; he was purely exhausted and resigned. "We were exactly where we were supposed to be, when we were supposed to be there. We took up position and waited for the convoy, but nothing moved in our direction."

Gradually the story unfolded, the pieces all fitting into place. The Pesh Merga had set an ambush for the convoy that defended Ser Genar. Despite being soaked through, hungry, and frozen they had all held their assigned places. Serwan joined them against doctor's orders and consequently wasn't strong enough to stand up to the tough conditions. After a while, he'd taken it upon himself to head to a factory where he might find bread and shelter.

"I warned him it was against orders," Ali explained. "I told him we had to hold our position, but he said he couldn't take it one more second." Ali pointed to one of the other Pesh Merga. "Didn't I tell him if he left we would see to it that he wound up in jail?"

Two of the attendant Pesh Merga nodded their agreement.

"Serwan knocked on the factory door, an old man came out, he talked to him briefly then went inside," Ali continued.

"Why didn't you go in after him?" Kurdo wanted to know.

"We waited for about twenty minutes, then I sent Ahsan to check out the building. The place was dark. He shouted for Serwan, but there was no answer."

"Why didn't you go inside?"

"By God, I heard voices speaking Arabic inside," Ahsan broke in. "I told you, but you didn't believe me," he shouted accusingly at Ali.

"Were you out of your mind, you coward?" Kurdo screamed.

"It wasn't that," Ali insisted. "I didn't want to take the risk. I wanted to go back and wait a few minutes."

"It was already too late," Ahsan scoffed. "We weren't back in our positions when heavy firing broke out."

From what I could piece together it seemed that when the firing broke out it was so strong that the Pesh Merga were taken by surprise and had no chance of returning the assault without endangering Serwan's life.

"What sort of cowards am I leading?" Kurdo scowled. "You knew Serwan was gone, you should have blown up the building with the enemy inside. You should be ashamed of yourself."

Ali opened his mouth to speak, but Kurdo cut him off. "Don't tell me you were thinking of Serwan. If he was inside a building with Arab speaking men, he was already lost."

"I did try the RBG, but the needle was stuck. It didn't work" Ali said sheepishly.

"Is that true?" Kurdo asked Ahsan. "Did you see him aiming at the building?"

"No, brother Nejmedin, I didn't. But it was very dark. Even so, he did give us the order not to shoot back, and he didn't say anything about the RBG not working."

Kurdo glared back accusingly at Ali. "You said the RBG didn't work, didn't you?"

"Yes! I tried both rockets, but they didn't go off."

Kurdo's eyes narrowed to slits. "Shalah," he turned to his closest aide. "Take the weapon outside and test it. Use both rockets."

Without a word of protest, Shalah grabbed the weapon and some ammunition and headed outside. An oppressive silence descended on the room as we all held our breath waiting for the outcome. Outside I could hear the sound of a distant battle, suggesting the surrounding areas were still under fire from various garrisons, but inside it was as silent as a tomb. Everyone present knew we were about to deal with our own very personal little battle.

BOOM! The sound of an explosion outside rocked the foundations of the humble little dwelling.

BOOM! A second explosion rocked the walls around us.

A moment later Shalah returned carrying the weapon in his left arm.

"There's nothing wrong with it," he said a little reluctantly. "But that doesn't mean a previous attempt to fire it didn't fail."

"Alright, alright, it's true," Ali admitted almost angrily. "I couldn't fire knowing Serwan was inside."

"You fool," Kurdo grimaced. "You cowardly fool! Can't you see that Serwan was already gone?"

"I made a decision in the heat of the moment. I thought it was better to go to the outskirts of the city and meet the other groups as planned, then we could return to the village together."

Apparently there had been heated debate as to the best course of action to take, and against Ali's wishes the majority decided to go back for Serwan planning to give the enemy troops inside an ultimatum: hand over our man, or be blown to kingdom come.

"It only took us ten minutes to get back to the factory," Ahsan explained. "But as we neared the yard I could feel it was already too late. All the lights were on and the old man was standing at the main door."

"Did you attempt to approach him?" Kurdo queried angrily.

"Of course! We told him to step forward and tell us what had happened to Serwan."

"And?"

"The old man spoke to us in a trembling voice. He said the enemy took Serwan away fifteen minutes before. He mumbled, 'poor boy, I hope they don't harm him'."

"Go on," Kurdo insisted.

"The old man explained when Serwan first knocked at the door, the enemy was already inside. He explained he couldn't warn Serwan because he would have been overheard. He said he tried to warn him off with hand signals, but Serwan didn't take any notice, or didn't understand. He said that Serwan just pushed inside and before he could say a word ten men had jumped on him and bound him tightly."

182

Kurdo closed his eyes for a heartbeat and turned his head away. "What else did the old man say?"

Ahsan looked at Ali regretfully before continuing. "They started to question Serwan, wanting to know how many Pesh Merga were outside. He told them ten times as many as we were. The enemy then called for backup and took Serwan to their headquarters."

"Did the old man tell you how many enemy forces were inside?"

"He said fifteen, and …"

"And?"

"They were Kurds."

Kurdo spat on the floor. Kurds fighting Kurds, it was the ultimate insanity. These were Kurds who had joined a mercenary team that fought alongside the Iraqi army against their own brethren, because they believed it afforded them a better chance of survival, and an increased share in the spoils upon victory. It was the very thing that Kurdo had deserted the army to escape from. My friend's eyes flashed fire. I knew the idea of killing his own brethren was abhorrent and shameful, but his wrath was brimming over with repugnant fury. I feared at that moment Kurdo could have been capable of almost anything.

"But their leader spoke to Serwan in Arabic," Ahsan added.

Kurdo sighed heavily and turned once again to his trusted aide. "Shalah, I want that old man in here by tomorrow."

Silently, Shalah nodded his agreement.

As Kurdo once again turned his attention towards Ali, I think everyone present took a collective breath.

"Give me your weapon," he ordered Ali.

The terrified Pesh Merga froze. Time itself seemed to freeze until another of the Pesh Merga took Ali's weapon from him and handed it to Kurdo. Slowly, and with very deliberately menacing movements, my friend caressed the weapon before pointing it at Ali. Nobody moved a muscle until with a sudden jerk Kurdo lowered the weapon again.

"You are relieved of duty until you stand trial in the morning," he announced impassively.

That night I tossed and turned in fitful and fretful sleepless dread. I thought about Serwan, and the torture he was almost certainly being subjected to. I thought about his father, and the torment that poor man would have to endure. And I thought about Ali, knowing that strictly speaking the punishment for his crimes would be death. Was my friend capable of carrying out such a punishment? How would I feel about him if the answer was yes? What would I do in his shoes? So many questions, and so few answers.

The following morning a committee was assembled in a nearby mosque, with both the French doctor and myself present. After three hours of intense and grueling questioning, no new facts were uncovered. I believe everyone in attendance reached the same conclusion, basically that Ali wasn't qualified to hold such an important position within the battalion, and that had he been able to think on his feet a little faster Serwan might still be with us today. At the very least the enemy soldiers, the treacherous Kurdish mercenaries, might have been captured or killed, which would have gone some way to placating this terrible loss. But none of these events transpired. Ali had failed in duty – failed terribly. His sentence ...

His sentence was to be stripped of his rank and dishonorably discharged. Other than that, he was free to go. We'd all seen enough bloodshed, and true to the person I knew him to be, Kurdo had no stomach for killing a fellow Kurd.

Serwan's father joined the trial about two hours into the proceedings. A respectful silence fell upon the mosque as the man who had just lost his son made his somber entrance to witness the Pesh Merga's form of justice.

"Come, kaloo," Kurdo beckoned him sympathetically ('kaloo' means 'uncle' – a term of affection). "Come, kaloo, and sit beside me. It is a hard day for us all today. We have lost kaka Serwan. He was left behind. My people have not behaved like men."

Serwan's father, who by all appearances was a strappingly healthy man, turned pale as a ghost. He said nothing. He simply watched stone-faced as the Kurdish Court completed their tribunal and handed down judgment.

Ashamed and disgraced, Ali left the building free and alive. I noticed Serwan's father follow him, wondering if the Pesh Merga's reprieve from a death sentence might be short-lived. But as I continued to watch it was obvious that all the father wanted to do was talk. They walked for hours. I could only assume the conversation might have been about Serwan's last free moments, or perhaps the father might be playing on Ali's guilt to convince him to attempt a rescue. In hindsight it mattered little. Five days later we received word that Serwan had been taken to the city of Kirkuk, tortured into signing a false statement, and then executed by firing squad.

CHAPTER FOURTEEN

At last we were on our way to cross Pira Magron en route to the 3rd battalion. What had begun as a pipedream to visit Kurdo on a social call had transformed into a call to arms where angels fear to tread. I kept glancing over to our young French friend, unable to fathom the images he'd (hopefully) one day return home with. As nightmarish images swirled through my vision, we began crossing the mountain with a complement of thirty men. Our mule, carrying medicines, dutifully followed along behind us. Once again it was raining heavily, but ironically we still needed water to drink. A bountiful supply presented itself in the form of a river we would later have to cross.

"Drink enough to get you to the other side of the mountain," a Pesh Merga instructed. "After this river there will be no more water until we reach the other side."

I looked up at the deluge falling from heaven and thought it was unlikely any of us would die from thirst. Besides, there was enough snow on the mountain to keep us all lubricated indefinitely.

"Drink," we were again ordered.

As instructed, we all took our fill of water before crossing the river that gave up its life-saving liquid to us. The road from there took us through a valley of huge rocks and down another ever-narrowing path. All the time Serwan's fate tumbled through my troubled mind. As soon as I was able to speak to Kurdo without the others hearing I had to clear the air.

"Do you think Ali was really responsible for Serwan's loss?" I asked quietly.

"Definitely," Kurdo snapped sharply in reply.

"Do you honestly believe he could have been stopped from seeking food and shelter? Or even that he could have been freed again later?"

"Yes, brother doctor, of course. Without discipline the Pesh Merga are nothing. Ali was not the right man to lead our people into action. But what's the use in talking about it now?"

He seemed – reflective. He wasn't the same man I'd met when I was a doctor in the general hospital, but then again none of us were. We'd all aged a hundred lifetimes in the past few months, our eyes and minds ravaged by sights and experiences that would haunt us to our graves.

"What is it?" I asked, sensing Kurdo was holding something back.

"Opportunists attract one another, like flies to honey."

"You mean Ali?"

"Exactly. Such people are more interested in holding onto their positions than fighting a revolution."

"I see. So you really believe Serwan could have been saved?"

"I do. Twice I was with Otman in a similar situation. On one occasion Otman went all the way to the window where firing was coming from, he snatched the weapons out of their hands, and threw a hand grenade into the room. On the other occasion it was the same thing, and we killed thirty-seven of the enemy."

"So in your mind, Ali should have attacked the building?"

"Of course! Serwan was already lost, we all knew it. Even if he did stand a chance, we would have had to attack the building, and if he didn't then we had to hit it with the RBG."

"But …"

I never did get the chance to finish that thought. Suddenly we came to an abrupt halt at a dead end of the valley where another mountain loomed before us. At this altitude the rain was transformed into snowflakes that might have been very picturesque on a Christmas card, but which proved an infuriating hindrance to mountaineers. There was no way the mule could join us on what was an almost vertical climb. The faithful beast-of-burden was duly sent on his way along with his owner via a longer route, planning to meet up with us again on the other side. Weapons had to be slung over our backs for it

187

was quite impossible to keep from plummeting to our deaths without using both hands to grip on.

At this dizzying height I genuinely felt as though I could reach out and touch the clouds, perhaps even heaven itself. I held onto that notion over the next hour or so that it took to reach the peak. After such a struggle to ascend to the zenith, I was quite surprised to discover the summit was perfectly level. In the summer months this would have been welcome, but in winter it merely facilitated the accumulation of snow, which was now almost three feet deep. I looked down, only just able to see my knees above the blanket of frosted precipitation beneath me. It was remarkable. Even though the temperature must have been far below freezing, I didn't feel cold. Perhaps it was a combination of exertion and adrenaline that kept me warm; certainly there was no shortage of fuel to keep the adrenaline pumping ...

"What the ...?" I suddenly gasped, seeing a pack of hungry wolves appear from nowhere.

"They're just hungry," one of the Pesh Merga said casually.

"For what?" I wanted to know.

"For whatever they can clamp their jaws around," he explained matter-of-factly.

I looked at the upper halves of my legs (the only halves visible) and thought they could present a thoroughly appetizing morsel for a hungry pack of wolves.

"They won't attack a group of thirty people," the Pesh Merga smiled.

"But what if one of us falls behind?" I inquired nervously.

"That would be bad," he replied simply.

I frowned.

Seeing my fear, Kurdo raised his rifle and fired off a few shots. The explosion of firepower sent the hungry canines running, but not very far, and not for very long. As soon as they realized we had caused them no harm, they were back.

"What about the mule and his owner?" I asked, reminding myself of our communication signals. Firing off a shot should have been an indication to return fire, letting us know he was well and could hear us. No such reply was received. All we could do was hope we reached the other side before nightfall, and pray that our mule and his storytelling owner could find a way of meeting us there.

Over the next two hours we lost track of one of the men in our group altogether, reaching a grisly total of three missing souls if one included our faithful mule and his master. Despite this fact we were past the point of no return. We had to push forward even though the storm was intensifying with every step we took. There was maybe an hour of daylight left. If we hadn't commenced our descent before darkness there was little doubt that most of us would have frozen to death. All the while I continued to fire off shots, hoping our missing companions would eventually reply. As each agonizing minute slipped by, my hopes slowly slipped away with them. And still we marched on.

There is an old adage; in fact there are several of them, such as, 'It is always darkest before the dawn', and 'look for the light at the end of the tunnel', and 'fortune favors the bold'. Stubbornly reminding myself that most clichés had a foundation in logic, and therefore refusing to give up hope entirely, I maintained my vigil of firing shots into the wilderness. Just as I thought I might be castigated for wasting ammunition I heard what I'd been waiting for – a reply! After all this time at first I thought it was just an echo. I fired again. The reply was swift and sure. Someone was alive! Our reunion must have seemed a little like a melodramatic scene from 'Doctor Zhivago' where two people jubilantly reunite in frozen wastelands with tears in their eyes. The storyteller from Azad literally leapt towards me.

"Brother doctor, I never thought we'd see each other again," he blurted, kissing me.

I hugged him like a long lost brother, for that was exactly what he was. I literally felt all the tense anxiety in his body leave him as I held him in my arms and he quietly slithered through my grasp, collapsing into the snow before me.

"Get up," I pleaded.

"I can't," he murmured weakly.

Everyone helped the poor man to his feet, dusted off the snow that had covered him, and he was given one of the Pesh Merga's coats to wear. If he could have cried, he would, but the dear storyteller was frozen solid and I suspect in shock.

Throughout this entire drama our French friend had remained unnervingly silent. I do believe at one point everyone had been given the option of keeping up the pace or being shot and left behind for the wolves. I guessed that would be sufficient motivation to keep everyone on their toes! The Pesh Merga, of course, had seen it all before, as had I. But what kept the French doctor so calm? It was a mystery never fully explained.

Darkness fell as we began our descent. The storm weakened and fog rolled over us like a warm welcoming blanket. I never thought I'd love fog! Like an affectionate caress we reveled in the embrace of our unearthly mantle, following each other blindly. It didn't occur to me for an instant that we might be on the wrong path, until ...

"My God!" Kurdo snapped abruptly. "This is the wrong village. It's probably full of mercenaries!"

That was not good! The village we'd stumbled into was directly on the highway between Dokan and Sul. Such areas were indefensible and routinely terrorized by the treacherous mercenaries. It was not unheard of for forces to move in, round up the locals, burn their houses, take all their livestock and grain, and leave a scene of utter devastation. But there was no way around it. All we could do was ready our weapons and move in.

Dogs started to circle us, as though they'd been taking lessons from their no-so-distant cousins, the wolves. They barked loudly, heralding the village's early warning system. Furtive glances were exchanged as we all wondered who would come out to greet us – friend or foe.

A smile! Oh yes, there was a God. The villagers were friendly. This was one area the mercenaries had not yet plundered. We were not only safe, but invited to stay. It was an attractive offer, but our final destination was still a long and laborious march away. We had to keep moving; after a quick visit to the mosque where we could clean up.

The next village we reached seemed deserted. The dogs were quiet, the lights were off – it felt like a cemetery. It wasn't that late, maybe eight or nine in the evening. So why was everything so still? The reason for the dark silence soon became apparent. It was our old friend – fear. What a sad and sorry state of affairs this was.

190

Nevertheless, one of the Pesh Merga found the local Party official and we were duly treated to the usual Kurdish hospitality.

At this point we would have just about sold our souls to get hold of a tractor to take us the rest of the way.

"There is one in town," we were advised by the local Party official. "But I don't think the owner will loan it to you."

"Nonsense," Kurdo quipped back. "Where is this owner? I want to see him."

Not wanting to argue with a Pesh Merga, the Party official disappeared and returned a short while later accompanied by a short, fat man in his sixties with a full mop of white hair.

"Have a seat, kallo," Kurdo said in a gentle and friendly manner.

The old man stubbornly remained standing.

"I understand you have a tractor."

"Yes I do, but ..."

Kurdo cut him off before he could continue his protest. "There are thirty Pesh Merga here who have to reach the 3rd battalion tonight. It's very important."

"I don't have enough gasoline for such a long journey," the old man complained. "And besides, the battery isn't strong enough."

"We will pay all your costs. And if you don't want to make the journey with us, we can send someone back with your tractor tomorrow."

"I'm very sorry, but ..."

"Brother," the Party official intervened. "These are our brave sons. You must help them."

"I can't," the old man stammered. "Our village is on the highway. I can't travel there with thirty Pesh Merga."

I could see the old man's point. If mercenaries turned up in this village and learned he'd lent assistance to the Pesh Merga his fate would be more horrible than anyone cared to contemplate.

"Don't force the man," I urged my companions.

"Brother doctor, you don't understand. If we were mercenaries this man would take us and not even request any form of compensation."

"He is a Kurd, and this is his war," Kurdo said icily, prompting the Party official to turn to one of his aides.

191

"Go and get one of this man's sons and tell him to have the tractor ready in fifteen minutes," the official barked, before turning back to the old man. "If you do not do your duty as a Kurd, you will walk with the Pesh Merga all the way to the 3rd battalion in bare feet! And when you return here I will see that you are put in jail!"

What had it come to? We were beginning to turn on each other.

Before long the aide blustered back into the room. "Brother! The women have hidden the old man's sons and wouldn't let us in."

The old man cowered, anticipating severe admonishment.

"What kind of people are you?" Kurdo growled at him. "What is the difference between you and a mercenary? Every day hundreds of Pesh Merga die to defend your freedom, and you – you ..."

"I support the revolution, brother," the old man insisted.

A knot formed inside my gut. I didn't like what I was hearing.

"I am not so sure of that," the official spat.

Kurdo began to circle the old man like a hungry shark. "If I were not a Pesh Merga I would shoot you on the spot and have your house burned to the ground."

"By God," the Party official added. "If we were mercenaries he would never dare refuse our request."

"That is our problem," Kurdo said soulfully. "We have never been hard with the enemy. If we had we would not have thousands of mercenaries among our people."

I found myself wondering about – everything. The Party official had accused the old man of collaborating with the mercenaries. Next time the mercenaries came to town this could cause grave problems. It was courageous indeed to risk such wrath. Then I thought about the courage of the hundreds of thousands among our people who were willing to do all that was humanly possibly to prevent Kurdistan from falling to its knees. Such courage amongst such insanity. Where was it all going to end?

When I had the opportunity to discuss these events with Kurdo at a later date he told me the Party official was a brave and decent man. As commander of the 4th Battalion, Kurdo received intelligence about tanks coming to the outskirts of the village and shelling without letup until the official agreed to present himself. Even before the war officially began, or rather reignited, these techniques were adopted.

192

Only once had the official gone to meet the tanks on the highway, and then only because the villagers demanded it as the mosque had been hit.

"What happened?" I gasped. "He really went out there?"

"Yes he did," Kurdo confirmed. "The military officer asked the usual questions and told him that every time they wanted to speak with him they would continue to hit the outskirts of the village until he showed up. They demanded cigarettes and tea, and they even had the gall to hand him propaganda material to distribute around the village. He threw the garbage in his fire while the tanks were still loitering on the outskirts."

It was easy to understand how a man's heart could be turned to stone against such a merciless backdrop of events. Meanwhile there was a situation brewing before my eyes. As Kurdo and I neared to the home of the old man we could hear women's voices begging the Pesh Merga not to take their father.

"Kurdo, what are we turning into? This is not how we behave," I begged.

"Desperate times call for desperate measures," he shot back stonily.

I watched as my friend headed towards one of the women, wondering what had become of the idealistic young man I'd met when I was in the general hospital.

"What is wrong, sister?" Kurdo asked.

"You tell me, kaka. They want to take my father and he has done nothing wrong."

"Not even the mercenaries treat us this badly," a second woman chimed in.

"I beg you," a third woman added her voice. "Please leave our father alone. He has done you no harm."

Their tearful pleas touched the heart of one of Kurdo's Pesh Merga, Mahommed.

"Perhaps you should think the matter over carefully before deciding to take the old man along," Mahommed suggested to Kurdo.

"I have," Kurdo growled back. "He's coming with us."

As we left all three women were crying, their tears mingling with the freshly falling rain. The old man stood his ground, refusing to

193

loan us his tractor, and Kurdo stood his, insisting the old man join us all the way to the 3rd battalion – on foot. I don't think a single word was exchanged during the sixteen-hour trek. The loudest utterances were our collective grimaces and scowls. We were all angry, and we were angry with everything. Angry with the situation. Angry with the old man. And angry with each other. Just plain angry.

The hills were muddy, the rain was heavy, and the mood was miserable. The old man walked alone, no doubt cursing us for bringing him along, and still the young French doctor passed no comment on anything. At one of our pit stops en route, where we paused for breakfast, our village host pleaded with Kurdo to free the old man, but still he stubbornly refused. Nothing about this felt right to me, a repugnant guilt was festering in my soul about the actions I was inextricably a part of. I had held Kurdo in such high esteem, it darkened my soul to see what he was becoming, and it enraged my mind knowing it was the fascist Ba'ath Party who brought this war upon us that drove my friend to dive to these depths. Nonetheless, whatever the reason, I was a part of this grim charade, and I couldn't shake the guilt of it. As if in manifestation of that guilt, my right knee began to grind.

With each step my bones crunched against one another uncushioned by any comforting cartilage between them. Each movement was sheer agony; although with all the walking I had done it shouldn't have been surprising that my cartilage was beginning to give way. Matters were improved none by the sub-zero temperatures and a violent wind lashing at our faces without let-up. Had it been just a little warmer I could have ridden a mule to save the immense anguish I experienced every time I placed one foot in front of the other, but with the weather the way it was if I had mounted a mule I would have frozen inside five minutes.

As soon as we reached the village of Seway I treated my ailment with occupational therapy; that is to say I attended to those who were far worse off than I in rebuke for any self-pity I'd indulged in. My French colleague assisted in the dispensary where we treated the usual stream of patients before heading to the prison where we also administered to the captured soldiers and mercenaries. The old man remained with us throughout our time this village. He never complained, in fact he never spoke at all. His silence spoke volumes. For three days we ate, slept and worked alongside one another, yet not once did he utter a syllable. Only when we were leaving Seway did Kurdo finally decide to send our reluctant traveling companion to Brigade headquarters, where I later heard he was detained for three days before being set free.

The battalion at Seway was planning an attack on the tanks and armored cars controlling the Dokan highway as we departed. This highway ran between Kirkuk and Sul, leading to the Dokan dam where ambushes were commonplace from both sides of the warring factions. By this dam of damnation, military vehicles and civilians alike were regularly blown from the face of the earth by mines, shelling, and low-flying jets. I have too many tragic memories of that highway – tragic for both sides – tragic for the whole Iraqi people. But this was war, and it was a war that had to continue until the tyranny of the Ba'ath regime and the Shah were obliterated from living memory. The fascist leadership of the central government had no regard whatsoever for the deprived peasants it forced into servitude under its military might. They routinely used the most underprivileged of their people to drive in civilian cars ahead of their convoys as human shields to clear the road ahead of any undetected mines. It was unconscionable, and unforgivable.

One of my dear friends was killed in an ambush on this highway. On the day he left for this duty he seemed to know he wasn't coming back. I recall him saying something along the lines of, "Kaka, this will be my last mission." Who knows what terrible foresight he'd witnessed, but whatever it was it proved to be correct. It had been a cold September morning when my friend and fifteen of his men arrived at an army outpost a little before sunrise. They watched and waited like stealthy predators, knowing the army's soldiers would be changing guards at the checkpoint outside Kirkuk come sunup. The team had scarcely taken up their positions when an armed car heaving with soldiers rolled in front of them, just a few meters away. The soldiers didn't stand a chance. They were no sooner out of their vehicle when all thirty were mowed down. It was normal procedure in these attacks to collect the enemy's weapons, a task which was completed in a matter of minutes. So hurried was the operation that when a head count versus weapons count was taken, the team realized they'd left one of the pistols behind. As firearms were as valuable to the fighting force as food and water, my friend offered to return and retrieve the missing armament.

Believing he need fear nothing, this man headed straight towards a surviving soldier who had crawled behind the wreckage for cover – armed with the missing weapon. A shot rang out, hitting my friend in the head and killing him instantly. On our continuing journey, my French colleague and our accompanying Pesh Merga came precariously close to this highway bringing all the memories of that fateful day flooding back. But life goes on; and the battle goes on. The battle of the Seway battalion had already commenced, and each sickening explosion reached across the distance between us ringing in our ears with crystal clarity. Artillery fell like rain, and in Kurdistan it certainly knew how to rain. Even after the battle was apparently over, and we reached the next village, there was no lull in the hostilities. We were forced to sit huddled in a humble dwelling of stones, wood, and mud as the village itself was shelled relentlessly. At any moment I was certain our roof would explode and that would be the end of all of us. All I could do was sit and wait for the inevitable. Glancing around the villagers beside me I didn't know whether to admire their bravery or castigate their stupidity. They could have built shelters. They didn't, believing to show fear was shameful.

By morning it was apparent that my maker had no desire to meet me just yet. We survived the night and marched on to the next village where we were not only greeted with a generous feast but, praise the powers that be, we were given a tractor to continue our journey. At this point my French colleague decided he had seen enough. He asked to be taken to a location from where he could return home. Many years later he contacted me again, sending me copies of the wonderful photographs he'd taken during his journey with us, congratulating my compatriots and I for the work we'd done with the people of Kurdistan. He went on to explain he'd terminated his experience with us believing he'd tempted fate once too often; another close call with death might well have been his last.

All of this taught me one thing – to be careful what you wish for. As an idealistic revolutionary who wanted to visit my friend Kurdo

196

and enter the real fighting to offer whatever support I could, I had put myself in harms way. I'd risked my life, which was selfish as there was no one else who would take over the running of the hospital in Azad. I'd put my French colleague in jeopardy. And perhaps worst of all, the experience had chipped away another little piece of my soul.

CHAPTER FIFTEEN

Back in Azad both the winter and the war continued with equal brutality. In the months that followed I treated more cases than I care to remember, but at least we were well-equipped with a good water supply, electricity, food, medicines, incredibly dedicated personnel, and a robust facility to operate from. With each new day my tired eyes witnessed more death, more destruction, and more despair than my mind could truly process. I could have turned inward and hardened my heart to the vast volume of violence around me, but something inside me said this wouldn't make me either a better person or a better doctor. Never once did I allow a case to become a statistic. Every life counted. Every person I saved was a triumph, every one I lost a tragedy. One in particular stands out vividly in my memory to this day.

I'd just finished my evening tour of the wards when a tall man with gray hair and beard was brought to me. He took me by the shoulders and tried to kiss me. I remember withdrawing, prompting him into a warm embrace instead.

"Brother doctor," he began in a cold hard tone, as though deliberately trying to mask a broken heart. "Please try to save my son. I have already lost three sons since the revolution started. He is all I have left."

"I will do all I can, kaloo," I assured him, trying not to show any signs of emotion myself.

It didn't take long for me to reach the conclusion that the young Pesh Merga was already dying. The older man gazed deeply into my eyes and began to weep.

"Come, come," I said, almost as though it was an order. "We don't have time for that now." Even as the words left my lips I could hear my own voice breaking with hopeless grief.

There was no mortal power that could have prevented his last son from passing. There were at least thirty holes in his body where mercenaries had machine-gunned him at close range. Had he ever had any chance of survival, which was doubtful, the six-hour journey to my hospital squashed it completely. The young man was riddled with injuries across his chest, abdomen and head. He was paralyzed, in a coma, and so cold it was possible to believe that rigor mortis had already set in. What did these people expect from me? I was not a God. I was just a man incapable of performing miracles; just a man who sometimes couldn't arrest wicked thoughts of selfishness, such as wondering why this boy couldn't just have died where he was shot. What was the point of wasting valuable medicines and precious time on a man who stood no chance of survival whatsoever? Even as that thought permeated my mind, I could see the poignant pleading in the father's eyes. Against my better judgment I began infusions and administered high doses of cortisone. Donors were cross-matched to assess whose blood type was suitable and the father was asked to wait outside.

Before the cross-matching was even completed, the seventeen-year-old Pesh Merga died. I sighed heavily, as though my own life force was so tired it too wanted to leave my body. With a somber expression and a steady step I went outside to talk to the boy's father. He took one look in my eyes and I knew I didn't need to speak.

"Kaka doctor, he is dead – my son is dead, isn't he?"

I bit my lower lip. "Yes, kaloo. He is dead. I am sorry. I did all that I could."

"We brought him in a coffin to you. We shall take him back in the same coffin," he said simply.

With that the father turned and left, a completely broken man, and he was not alone. It had been the final straw for me too. That night I did something I had not done since taking up this assignment. I reached for a bottle of alcohol, intending to consume every last drop. And I cried.

I cried and cried until I thought my sides would burst.

I cried until I thought the rains in heaven couldn't compete with my outburst.

I cried and cried in the futile hope that in some way this would exorcise my demons, but such demons can never be exorcised; they live on in the mind for all eternity.

∞∞

To all beginnings there will be an end, so they say. But a revolution is a circle, a never-ending spiral that repeats and repeats on itself. The circle itself is a symbol of infinity, of perpetuity, of time without end, and the very word 'revolution' mirrors these physical facts. I didn't know if I could ever go back to living a normal life, whatever that meant. I didn't even know if there was a normal world still thriving outside the pitiless horror that had become my existence. What I did know was that as long as there was life there was hope, no matter how distant the illusive glimmer of that hope might be. Despite everything that had happened to these people they were not close to giving up; they would rather fight to the very last man, woman and child than surrender to the devilish dictatorship that ruled in Baghdad. If ever I saw the personification of their gritty resolve to survive, I saw it in my next tragic patient.

A young man of eighteen was brought to me so badly burned that his body resembled the charcoal in the smoldering embers of my fire. Paralyzed from childhood, the man had been caught in an inferno after an artillery shell had hit their home exploding a gas can. He was brought to me by his older brother in a prophetic coffin suffering third-degree burns over sixty-percent of his body. His skinny little legs were like matchsticks, burned out matchsticks. Beyond any normal measure of human endurance he fought for every last moment of life. We cleaned his wounds and assigned one dresser to look after this patient exclusively, even knowing his chances were slim at best. I truly couldn't believe my ears a few days later when the dresser told me the man had begun to eat.

"Hama Amin," I cheered, rushing to his side. "What would you like to eat today?"

"I would like to eat a whole chicken all to myself," he replied without any hesitation.

I couldn't help but smile. What a rare blessing that was, to feel permitted and able to smile.

"If a chicken is what you want, then a chicken you shall have," I beamed.

"No, brother doctor," his brother chimed in. "We have no money with us. We can't afford a chicken. It isn't …"

"The money doesn't matter," I said softly. "Seeing your brother is able to eat is a joy for us all. In fact I will give you some money from our budget to buy a chicken. You go and get it and take it to the kitchen. Tell Karim to cook it well with lots of soup."

I handed him a few pounds. "Go on, it's alright," I assured him, noticing he was looking at the money as though it might burn a hole in his hands.

"Thank you, brother doctor," he gushed, rushing off to purchase his brother's meal.

The following morning I hurried to the burn victim to see if he'd like another chicken.

"No thank you," the man said modestly. "I still have plenty. My brother refused to share it with me."

I looked accusingly at his brother. "You eat alongside him. We can always get another chicken. Besides, if you leave it too long it will spoil and be wasted."

"Yes, brother doctor," he answered as though he was a schoolboy receiving punishment.

The vigil at the young burn victim's bedside persisted as up to fifty centimeters of snow fell on our rooftop nightly. The guards assigned to the hospital worked tirelessly to shovel it away, but each night a fresh layer descended as though mocking our efforts. I sustained my duties, regardless of inclement weather, visiting my wards and attending to my patients' needs, until one morning the burn victim called to me again.

"Brother doctor," he said in an almost conspiratorial tone.

"Yes, Hama Amin. What is it?"

"Brother doctor," he whispered. "I will need some new clothes to go home in. Mine were all burned in the fire."

"Of course. No problem. I shall arrange for it," I fumbled.

His brother looked up at me sadly. I tried not to meet his gaze, but he wouldn't be dissuaded. He followed me out of the ward, leaving me no chance of escape.

"My brother will be leaving soon?" he demanded of me.

"Yes."

"He will leave to go home?"

I turned to meet the brother's wretched gaze. "You will be able to take him home," I said simply.

"Alive?"

I bowed my head. "The chance of a victim surviving third-degree burns to sixty-percent of his body would be slim at best, even in the most modern of hospitals."

"I see," he stammered, tears beginning to well in his eyes.

"It really is nothing short of a miracle he's done as well as he has," I tried to sound cheerful. "But he's not eating any more..." I shrugged expansively.

"I understand," the brother sobbed.

I watched him turn and walk inside with the weight of the world on his shoulders. A few days later I watched again as he placed his dead brother in the same coffin he had arrived in. I went on watching as he tied the coffin to his mule and began the journey to take the charred little body home, just as he'd promised. I watched until they became but a spec on the distant horizon before disappearing forever behind the hills of the vineyards.

∞∞

My fourteen months in Azad were like one long, bitter, cloud-covered day. As they neared their end, and the promise of spring became tantalizingly close, I had to make a trip to Pen Jewin for fresh supplies. My friend Kurdo said he would take a car to the village. Both his company and the transport were warmly welcomed, but I was having difficulty understanding his mood. He seemed twitchy with restlessness yet profoundly sad at the same time. Cars were not supposed to travel until after dusk, as the roads had become a long chain of military garrisons, so when he demanded our driver leave immediately I was shocked.

"Kaka, it's against orders," the driver told him.

"I don't care," Kurdo snapped back. "We have urgent business in Pen Jewin. We have to leave immediately."

"But we have strict orders from the Party not to go through until after dark."

"Kurdo," I pleaded with him. "You can't be serious."

"Of course I'm serious," he scowled. "You're not afraid are you, brother doctor?"

"Of course I'm afraid," I almost shouted. "It's madness! It's suicide!"

Although I hadn't realized it yet, suicide was exactly what was on Kurdo's mind. He had lost his hope. Any faith he'd ever had in the leadership of the Movement had long since perished alongside the many souls we'd seen lost. He welcomed death. In death at least there was freedom, a freedom he no longer believed he would find in life.

"I cannot take the responsibility," the driver told him.

"I'll take the responsibility, you coward!"

"Kurdo," I gasped.

"You will have to talk to the transportation official," the driver insisted.

"Fine," my friend grimaced in reply.

I have no idea how he did it, but somehow Kurdo convinced the official to let us take the car, with a land-rover following behind. As we pulled out from the leafy cover of our tree-lined canopy and headed further and further down the road towards the mountains, my heart began pounding so fast I thought it might explode from my chest. No one spoke, not one single word, as we ventured unerringly deeper into enemy territory. If memory serves, I think I did try to speak on several occasions, but no words would come out. Even though I couldn't see my own complexion I'm quite certain I was the same pale shade of gray as the driver. We were all quite literally sick with fear, knowing full well that one single blast from a tank would have blown us into oblivion. What made Kurdo behave this way? At the time I couldn't understand it. I was committed to saving life, all life, any life, at any cost. The very notion that anyone could choose to end a life for no reason was incomprehensible to me.

Again my maker didn't seem to have any interest in meeting me that day. Perhaps I'd done something to offend Him? This is not to say that our journey was without incident. With the warming sun melting the heavy snow our roads had become muddy bogs. In such conditions, it didn't take long for us to come across a vehicle hopelessly stuck in the mire.

"Stop and help them," Kurdo ordered.

"Kaka, I can't. We'll be destroyed," the driver shot back with an urgent sense of self-preservation.

From the land-rover behind I heard Ahmed shouting his opinion. "They are brothers. We have to stop to lend assistance."

"That's right," Kurdo agreed. "They're just civilians, and they need our help."

"I'm not going back, no matter what," the driver insisted. "You are wearing the khaki of the Pesh Merga and carrying weapons."

I couldn't stand it any longer. I opened the door and stepped outside for some fresh air while they continued screaming at each other. I judged I'd be safer outside in any event. If we were targeted, the army would aim for the vehicle not the lone man aimlessly wandering outside it. A moment later Kurdo followed me, his trusty Kalashnikov firmly by his side. The closest military outpost was only a kilometer away, perched strategically on the mountain from where we could easily have been spotted with a pair of binoculars. Carrying a weapon was yet another invitation for death, should Kurdo be spotted. I knew it. He knew it. He did it anyway. And I said nothing. Somewhere in the bowels of my being I knew any plea from me would fall on deaf ears, and likely only start another argument which could attract unwelcome attention

Happily it didn't take long to free the civilian car from the molasses of goo. We were duly thanked, in return for which we were ceremoniously gracious and promptly headed the hell out of there as fast as we could travel. We didn't stop again until we reached the relative safety of a teahouse in a little village off the main road. The traditional tea, bread and yogurt was distributed, all of which I consumed while looking curiously towards Kurdo.

"Did you notice anything strange out there?" he asked me in Arabic, knowing we were the only two in the group who could understand Arabic.

"You mean aside from the fact that I was scared to death?"

"I mean about Mustafa." (Mustafa was one of Kurdo's aides.)

"Mustafa? What about him?"

"When he went to pull the car out he left his weapon behind."

"So?"

"A good Pesh Merga never leaves his weapon behind when going into action."

"Action? I'd hardly call helping a few stranded civilians 'action'!"

"I have been watching Mustafa. He is scared."

"So am I," I snapped back, raising my eyebrows.

By this time Mustafa was looking at us. He might not have spoken Arabic, but he could hear his name being mentioned clearly enough.

"Mustafa," Kurdo turned to him, speaking in his native tongue. "Have I ever mistreated you in any way?"

"Never, kaka Kurdo."

"Then why did you leave your weapon behind out there? A good Pesh Merga is never parted from his weapon, not even in sleep."

"I didn't think it was necessary."

"What do you mean 'not necessary'? Aren't we at war? What is a Pesh Merga worth without his weapon?"

"I am sorry, kaka Kurdo. I made a mistake."

"Made a mistake," Kurdo echoed mockingly.

My dear, troubled friend would not be pacified. He sat down and wrote a long letter, put it in a suitable envelope, and handed it to Mustafa.

"Take this letter to the brigade headquarters. Give it to the commander and wait there until I return."

Mustafa scowled at the letter. He well knew the intent sealed inside. To be assigned to a headquarters was nothing short of becoming a servant, reduced to the most menial of labors such as dishing out food, bringing water, and acting as a cleaner. There was nothing more insulting or humiliating for a Pesh Merga.

We remained in that teahouse until eight in the evening. It was the end of the road for our driver, so we'd made arrangements to meet up with two villagers and their mules. When they didn't turn up we moved to another teahouse, which had a reputation for being open all hours, behind the Jawarta mountain. To our surprise, it was closed. Having traveled so far we thought it might at least be worth trying to knock on the door. Our audacity was rewarded by the shuffling footsteps of an old man who granted us shelter but was reluctant to use his dwindling supply of wood to heat the stove for tea. This should have been a sign. Teahouses were famed for their hospitality in any circumstances. Nothing was right. Nothing was right about anything. My friend was suicidal. My nerves were completely shattered. And to top it off this teahouse was utterly cold and unfriendly. There was nothing to eat, and we had to spend the night on a cold, hard floor with mice running all over us. The owner didn't even have a cat to keep the little vermin away.

Drifting into a restless sleep I thought back to the time I first met Kurdo. I saw the idealistic spark of a blossoming revolutionary in his youthful eyes. I recalled the laughter and camaraderie we'd shared. My mixed-up mind leapt in all directions, one minute seeing myself treating Kurdo's wounds as he lay in my hospital in Azad, the next thanking him for his generosity as he gave me my much needed generator, the next being perched up on a hilltop watching him go into battle to take the city of Sul. We had been through so much together, and achieved so much, I couldn't believe thoughts of self-termination were entering his mind. Those bright enthusiastic eyes I'd once known were now bitter, hardened, and glazed. This war had left his spirit desolate and his soul plundered. Could anyone find their way back from the depths of such despair?

As dawn broke over the horizon the missing mules and their owners arrived with profuse apologies. They explained they'd spent the night in Jawarta itself because their loyal and hard-working animals were worn out and needed feeding. I could certainly sympathize with that; exhaustion and hunger were qualities we all shared in common. No doubt the mules had enjoyed a far more comfortable night than we'd contended with, not that there was much competition on that score. Certainly they would have been fed better, anything more than nothing would have been an improvement after all. However, I didn't begrudge them their comfort or their food; how could I begrudge such basic necessities to the faithful beasts-of-burden who were forced to endure more than their share of the hardship of this land? On balance, in retrospect, I was pleased they'd had a good night.

It was raining – again – of course. And I'd no sooner returned to foot trudging when my knee started to give me terrible grief once more. I soldiered on as best I could as we climbed more mountains and descended into more charming little villages nestled in picturesque valleys. At least in the rest of the teahouses we stopped at we were treated to the more traditionally warm hospitality I'd become accustomed to. Crossing one particularly magnificent landscape, amidst beautiful babbling brooks set against the awesome grandeur of Kurdistan's ageless and rugged mountain ranges, my knee gave up altogether. There was nothing for it; I was going to have to ride a mule. Even if I froze to death hiking up hill and down dale it would have to be an improvement on the excruciating pain I could no longer either ignore or endure.

Inch by inch we closed in on our target like unwavering homing pigeons or salmon swimming upstream against powerful currents, driven by a potent primordial yearning to return to their spawning ground. Only death would sway the salmon or the homing pigeon from their destination; only death would sway us. The last three hours of the journey presented us with flat terrain, which on the face of it seemed like good news. But the heavy rains had transformed otherwise green meadows into a veritable sea of mud. Still we continued. Pen Jewin was close.

Why was it I always seemed to arrive in Pen Jewin caked in mud and exhausted? I sometimes wondered if the locals had come to think of me as some kind of chocolate-covered, bespectacled, snowman. When we landed in this bustling city of thriving trade I wanted to scream, "Don't you people realize what we've just been through?"

For long moments I studied the populous scurrying around like industrious little termites building a palatial mound to dwell in. The teahouses and restaurants on both sides of the narrow street were crammed with patrons. All the shops were distended with goods. It seemed to be a thriving metropolis of endeavor, yet when I looked a little closer something was out of place. Despite the apparent hive of activity the faces of the people betrayed the reality of the situation. Those faces were pale, weak, and very, very frightened.

"We're losing this battle," I mumbled to myself.

"Perhaps it is better," Kurdo responded.

I looked at him quizzically.

"At least if we lose, the war ends," he explained. "Look at these people. How much more do you think they can handle? We are going about this all wrong, and a greater power is punishing us for our blunder."

"Isn't time on the side of the revolution?" I asked.

"Sometimes I think we are a football team without a captain," he grizzled back, wandering off to attend to some personal business he claimed to have.

For the next three days I haggled with the newly-appointed young doctor of the area who'd been put in charge of handling supplies. I might as well have been negotiating with an African aardvark. This child had no concept of what the real war was like. He'd never crossed the dark mountains into the real Kurdistan to experience the full horror of our war first hand. Even with my most diplomatic, charming, and logical arguments he refused to give me more than a month's supply of medicine and money. My only option to secure further supplies was to head to the other side of the border to meet with the department chief. It seemed like a plan.

CHAPTER SIXTEEN

Did I say it seemed like a plan? On the other side of the border I received no more joy than I had with the aardvark. Had the whole world gone mad? It was a stupid question. Of course it had! People in these border towns had no concept of what life was like in the interior of Kurdistan. I needed to vent my anger. Where was Kurdo?

I hurried back to Pen Jewin, hoping to find my friend and bend his ear about the imbeciles I was forced to contend with. Where was he? I couldn't find him anywhere. Even his aides didn't know where he'd disappeared to. I wasn't about to return to Azad without him, so I wrote a letter explaining I would have to remain in Pen Jewin for a few more days and sent it home with the mules and their owners. Over the days that followed a crucial turning point occurred in the war; an event set in motion at a meeting held thousands of miles away behind closed doors in Algiers.

While I remained in Pen Jewin the heads of governments from several of the oil-producing countries, including Iran and Iraq, were called to clandestine talks. The leadership of the Kurdish Movement was not informed, and not invited. It was March, 1975, when hard bargaining by the friendlier countries in the region convinced Iran and Iraq to apparently settle their differences. No direct reference was made to the Kurdish 'problem', as such. Rather it was concluded that border conflicts would be settled according to old treaties and each country would therefore respect the sovereignty and borders of the other. Each State would refuse entry to intruders from the other side in order to prevent sabotage and subterfuge from enemy operatives against the other country. In other words, the Kurds were stranded – cut off from important supply and support channels to the revolution. Barzani, the Kurdish leadership, was left with no option but to comply without objection or consultation. The moment the Algiers agreement was signed, Iran withdrew and forbade any assistance to the Kurdish Movement. Our leadership was cut loose like a lone dinghy in a ferocious tempest in the middle of an uncharted ocean.

Close observers of the situation concluded the Kurdish leadership now had one of three choices:

Surrender,

Accept the so-called 'amnesty', or

Fight to the death.

This boiled down to a choice between betraying everything we believed in, as well as the memories of those who had given up their lives for the cause, and facing the certainty of yet more violence and oppression, or continuing the battle and confronting greater grueling hardships than we'd already endured. Some choice!

This battle had already known the wrath and ferocity of fourteen long years of war. I didn't believe there was any power on earth that could stop it now. Even without Teheran's aid, the Movement's leadership considered there was sufficient finances available to keep the frenzied flames of fury fanned for many years to come. There were stock piles of ammunition. There were sixty-thousand Pesh Merga prepared to give their all. And there were forty-thousand square kilometers of freed land suitable for maintaining the struggle. But perhaps more importantly than any of this was the will of the people.

There were many who continued to cry, "We fight for victory. We will never surrender!" Yet as I walked the narrow streets of Pen Jewin, listening to the radio broadcasts from Baghdad and Teheran, I couldn't help but notice the people looked confused. Everyone had a different interpretation of the agreement. There were expressions of hopeful expectation in some eyes, a yearning for peace at any cost in others. Personally I had grave misgivings about the situation. From my point of view Kurdistan had become totally dependent on outside help, without it the struggle seemed impossible. I gazed sadly upon a people who'd believed this battle would be over before the cruel winter set in, yet spring was beginning to bloom and still we were at war. Of course these were the same people who'd believed in the fairytales of modern tanks, big rockets, and even their own modest air force.

For the most part what I saw were people who wanted peace at any cost – whatever the cost. Their spirit was broken and their confidence crushed. I understood, I understood only too well, but how high is the cost of peace if you're trading in your weapons for the stale bread of slavery? How could one find peace in the arms of a tyrannical enemy? Why would anyone volunteer to become a refugee in their own land?

As I searched for the answers, I also searched for a tractor to take me back to Azad. And I searched for something else – Kurdo.

Before long a telegram was sent from the leadership of the Movement to all battalions under their control. The key word was 'truce'. The notice was dry, brief, and precise. For the following two weeks there would be a truce. Pesh Merga were to stop all activities, but they were to maintain battle-readiness and strike back if hit. All of Kurdistan celebrated, firing thousands upon thousands of rounds into the sky, unaware of concessions the Ba'ath Party had made to Iran. I was still in Pen Jewin when the Movement's propaganda machine swung into action. The word on the streets was suddenly that our struggle was noble and just and would continue regardless of consequences. What the Shah's and the Ba'athist's regimes said was irrelevant. This was a peoples' war and it would continue until the aspirations of the people had been achieved.

The Movement rationalized their decision by saying they could cut costs by reducing the number of active Pesh Merga, culling the old, the weak, and the worn-out. The thousands of people who had joined the Movement just a year ago could return to their homes. People began to believe they could stand alone, unaided by the much-hated Iranian establishment, and maintaining their commendable confrontation against the fascist tyranny in Baghdad to save all Iraqis from their brutal rule. More madness. Everywhere I looked it was madness. But perhaps the greatest madness of all was my own decision to make a stand and remain on until the bitter the end. I had come to serve, and while my service was still required, in Kurdistan I was going to remain. I had no idea how we could win this conflict without external assistance, but there was no way I was about to turn and run now.

The days of the truce ticked by quickly. If I was going to make it back to Azad I had to find a tractor, but every corner I turned was a dead end. My faithful assistants, Serwan and Diman, had both joined me in Pen Jewin. Neither one wanted to return to Azad. As bad as conditions were before, it was plain to see they were about to take a whole new slide downhill. I couldn't argue with Diman, he had a large family to care for. But Serwan was young, and the most skilled dresser I'd worked with. Losing him would be like cutting off both arms. It took a great deal of debate, but eventually I convinced him to return with me. Perhaps I was condemning him to death – or worse – but I couldn't cope with the thought of not having him by my side.

And where was Kurdo? In all the time I spent in Pen Jewin searching high and low for a tractor, there was no sign of him.

Azad – would I ever see it again? Would it survive this new onslaught? Even before this unholy alliance between Iran and Iraq, no doctor had been prepared to serve in my beloved Azad, yet somehow I had managed to make it work. It was true I hardly had a hundred percent survival rate, but the track record I had succeeded in achieving was admired across the Movement. I couldn't bare the thought that it had all been for nothing. I had to get back. I needed a tractor!

A plan was already forming in my mind to move the hospital as soon as I returned. As well protected as we were, relatively speaking, with a new round of hostilities I knew I couldn't protect my staff and patients in their present location any longer. I would move the hospital behind a nearby giant mountain, one that was covered with snow even in the summer. However, if I didn't find a tractor soon there would be no hospital to move. If my most loyal and trusted companions, Serwan and Diman, were willing to turn away, it was doubtful any of the personnel back in Azad would remain for long without my persuasion. They would soon be realizing that salaries and leave were a thing of the past. Trips across the border to spend rare free time with the exquisite horses of Karmanschah would be no more. Every meager little pleasure we'd created for ourselves was about to be stripped away as though it never existed at all.

In Pen Jewin the situation was becoming chaotic. Officials were trying frantically to ascertain who were the most able bodied, the most honest, and the most prepared to fight. Confusion reigned supreme. It seemed everything was breaking down as the truce ticked methodically and unwaveringly towards an end. And still there was no tractor – and no Kurdo!

March 14th, 1975. Success! A tractor! The brigade headquarters sent word to me that four tractors would be leaving Pen Jewin shortly, heading in my direction. I was further advised there was enough room to load all my supplies, if I hurried. Without needing to be told twice, I raced towards the dispensary where my provisions were stored, and sent Serwan off to buy a plastic cover for the medicines (as naturally it was raining again). At 11am precisely the four tractors, heavily laden with Pesh Merga and fully loaded trailers, pulled out in convoy towards the rugged mountain ranges. Sinister-looking black clouds loomed ahead. As one could see images in flames, I saw faces in those clouds; ominous omens of dread sneering at me through dark fluffy masks. I looked away, gazing back one last time upon the disoriented and poignantly melancholy faces of the people in Pen Jewin. It was time to go, time to make my final stand, and I had to leave despite the fact that there was still one nagging question gnawing at me – where the hell was Kurdo?

As we rolled towards our date with destiny my mind drifted back to the many hours I'd spent with Diman. We'd shared tragedies and triumphs, laughter and tears, we were more than brothers, more than best friends, and suddenly I had a sinking feeling in the pit of my stomach that I'd never see him again. Farewell dear friend. You have been more special to me than you are ever likely to know.

Serwan and I were perched on the third of the four tractors, watching the city of Pen Jewin disappearing from our sight; a spec in the distance that vanished as we rolled behind the first of the mountains we had to pass. Although busy and crowded, Pen Jewin was shrouded in a cloud of lonely isolation, its fragile people capable of being blown away like leaves before an angry wind.

"Do you think we'll ever see it again?" Serwan asked, as if reading my thoughts.

"Who knows," I shrugged. "Maybe."

"Do you really believe we're doing the right thing, going back?"

"It's our duty. Those people have needed our help for fourteen years, and especially over the last fourteen months. But they need it now like they've never needed it before."

Serwan didn't reply. We both knew this was a critical episode in the history of the Kurdish people. For the first time they were truly on their own, and to stand alone is perhaps the harshest challenge anyone can ever have to face. We remained in individual silent reflection right up until the moment when the first tractor inevitably became bogged. It took us half an hour to free it from a quagmire of sludge, and make the road passable for the other three. It was clear we wouldn't survive the journey over high, snow-covered, muddy mountains. The only other option was the longer route across smaller muddy hills, which also meant crossing rivers of surging furious waters.

On first attempt tractor one faired quite well, even though the tributary almost covered its huge wheels. The second beast didn't travel as well. Its engine packed up midstream. The third became wedged in the riverbed. Only the fourth managed to follow the good example of the first by making it all the way to the other side. Stuck on the third tractor with Serwan, I really did question the wisdom of my insane decision to put myself through all this again. But there I was, and there was no going back now.

It didn't take long for the drivers of the two surviving tractors to attach thick, steel ropes to their two ailing cohorts and drag them back to terra firma. These drivers were skilled and experienced, and I doubted if they could be diverted by the fires of hell itself.

The following two days tested our fortitude time and again. One of the trailers hit a rock and tumbled over. One of the tractors had a battery that was spluttering its last breaths. This meant it could only move between the others at night as it didn't have enough juice left to fire both its engine and its headlights. I lost count of how many times we seemed immovably lodged in slimy black goo, the menacing mud that refused to loosen its grip on our steel-clad steeds. We became expert at unloading and loading the trailers to lighten the load and hence enable our escape. And then we ran out of fuel!

"I'm sorry," the driver said to us. "This is as far as I can take you. I should have had enough fuel for two more trips, but the damn mud has burned it all out."

"Well naturally," I thought out loud. What else? Surely the journey would be no fun at all if it wasn't fraught with more trials and tribulations than we could possibly anticipate! There was nothing else for it. We had to head to the nearest village to beg, steal or borrow some mules, and we had to get our supplies to safety at all costs.

Could we find mules? Of course not! The best solution we were able to come up with was to manually relocate the supplies to a nearby deserted schoolhouse we came across, and head back to Azad on foot. From there we could find mules to send back for the medicines. It was a long road home, and all the way it seemed our decision to make a stand to the bitter end put us in a firm minority. A veritable exodus was flooding the thoroughfare, all heading the other way. Serwan made one comment, and chose not to mention it again.

"They're all heading to safety before the war starts again."

CHAPTER SEVENTEEN

Returning to Azad after a three-week absence it was immediately apparent this was not the same place I'd left. All the city dwellers who had joined the Movement, perhaps thinking they would return home after a victorious triumph to greater privileges, were leaving. Azad no longer glowed with the warm, welcoming generosity of spirit I had known. The villagers were despondent, dismal, and rejected. Children who, despite the war, had once played in the little paths that wound their way intricately around the township no longer lifted our morale with the carefree sound of their laughter.

There was a crushing atmosphere of nothing left to fight for – and nothing left to fight with. Yet I wondered where the deserters were running to. Every road led directly into the waiting arms of the enemy. Their best hope was to accept the so-called amnesty – an offer of fifty pounds together with a promise of their old jobs back if they surrendered their weapons. All because a treaty was signed between countries that had no interest in the plight of the Kurdish people; a treaty signed on foreign soil thousands of miles away in the supposedly neutral country of Algiers. Madness! How could anyone be so easily duped?

It was obvious I was too late. I felt lonely, cheated and betrayed. Even the brigade officials were leaving town.

"Look at those cowardly bastards," Serwan scowled.

Everything I'd created was disintegrating before my eyes, but even so I couldn't find it in my heart to chastise these people. They were frightened and confused, and who could blame them? A revolution is perhaps the hardest of all wars to fight because only with the support and will of the people can it be fought. No one is conscripted or drafted to fight a revolution; they come willingly, or they don't come at all.

"Cowards," Serwan growled again.

"If that is how you feel," I said slowly, "perhaps it is better they leave now than become a burden on us later."

He didn't answer me.

We walked into the local Party headquarters almost unnoticed. Only one man acknowledged us. Sherko, a comrade through much of this horror, looked pale and tired, but as soon as he spotted us he jumped to his feet and ran towards me.

"It's all finished, brother doctor, isn't it?" The downhearted and disillusioned man hugged me until he nearly squeezed the life out of me.

"What are you talking about, kaka?"

"The telegram from Barzani. It's true isn't it, brother doctor?"

"What telegram?" I asked, totally mystified.

"Yesterday afternoon a telegram signed by Barzani arrived at Brigade headquarters."

"Saying the fight would continue?" Serwan asked, almost as though it was a statement.

"No, kaka Serwan. The telegram says the struggle is over. We are to drop all our weapons at once. We have been given a choice of surrendering to the Iraqi government or moving to Iran."

"This can't be true," I shouted angrily. "When we left Pen Jewin everyone was preparing to continue the fight. I have brought enough supplies back with me to last for six months."

"I pray you are right, brother doctor. But the Pesh Merga lieutenant has received orders to blow up the brigade's ammunition depots at noon today."

"We have to stop him," Serwan blurted.

"It's no use," Sherko insisted. "Twice he received the instructions, and twice he said he would rather commit suicide than carry them out. So far he's continued to refuse, even though there have now been four telegrams from headquarters."

My head was swimming. My legs completely buckled underneath. I slumped into the nearest chair not caring, not even realizing that I was still in my muddy wet clothes. A sea of faces whirled through my

217

mind; all the parents who had lost their children; the sixteen-year-old mother who'd saved her infant and lost her arm, the other Serwan who'd been tortured and executed. And how many now would commit suicide believing this was the only escape left? How many more would seek revenge by committing acts of terrorism, killing still more? And where the blazes was Kurdo?

"Where are Hama and Darwish?" I asked Sherko quietly, thinking of all the loyal people who'd worked so tirelessly by my side.

"They have gone to brigade headquarters to find out if it's really true."

Someone in the background piped up, "I believe it is true, kaka doctor. I tell you, we've been sold out!"

"Perhaps the army broke our code and telegrammed in the name of Barzani," Sherko suggested.

"Daydreams, kaka!" Serwan snapped back.

"As I sit here I swear to you, when we left Pen Jewin there were not even rumors about surrender," I assured everyone. "I have orders to transfer the hospital to a safer location."

Silence descended on the room. These poor, disheartened people were being swallowed whole by fear and mistrust, and I had still worse news for them.

"I don't think we can count on any salaries in the future," I told them reluctantly. "But I still hope everyone makes the right decision."

"Are you asking us to stay, kaka doctor?" one of the villagers inquired.

"Yes I am," I said firmly.

"By God," the villager stood up shouting. "If kaka doctor is prepared to stay until death, then we should stay with him!"

"Huh! So much for thinking you've broken the will of the people," I mumbled under my breath in Arabic, thinking of the central government.

"Anyone who decides to stay shouldn't do so because of one man," I said out loud.

I understood only too clearly that the people of Azad were driven by tribal loyalties that were nearly as old as time itself. If the head of a tribe told them to jump into a ball of fire, they would have done so without hesitation or apprehension. As many had come to see me as a de facto tribal leader, I feared I had but to ask and they would follow where I led. I wanted them to stay, and to support the hospital that would be so vital to whatever lay ahead, but I wanted them to make that decision of their own free wills, because they believed it was right, not because I told them to.

It was 11:30am when we received word that Hama and Darwish were on their way back from headquarters. Eager to hear their news, whatever it was, we rushed outside towards the last hill in the village where we could meet them. At first I didn't notice it had stopped raining. Bright warm rays of sun were valiantly fighting through the thick gloomy rain clouds that stubbornly refused to dissipate. Was this a positive sign, a cosmic prophecy that even the darkest clouds cannot persist forever? My raw nerves tingled with anticipation as a promise of tomorrow hung in the air.

There they were! I spotted my two friends in the middle of a large group who had all demanded answers from headquarters. Oh no, was that rain I could see? No, not rain – tears. Some of those people were crying, and all of them wore undisguised depression as shrouds upon their faces. We didn't require the hollow series of questions and answers that followed. The outcome was obvious. But we went through the motions anyway.

"What's the news?"

"Unchanged. Drop and destroy all weapons."

"Are you sure it's from Barzani?"

"Definitely."

"Kaka, we are finished."

Those last words came from the Party official himself, as he turned and walked towards the nearest stream to wash his face. When he looked back he was weeping.

In among the crowd I noticed a tall man in a black overcoat carrying ten packets of Kalashnikov bullets.

"What's he doing?" I whispered to Hama.

"You remember him, he's the mercenary who was discharged from hospital a month ago and sent to the prison at headquarters."

"I remember him well enough, but what's he doing here, and with bullets?"

"The prison's been opened, and all mercenaries told to go home."

"But how did he get all those Kalashnikov bullets?"

"The Brigade's ammunition room was opened to the people. They were told they could take what they wanted before the whole lot is destroyed at noon." Hama looked at his watch. "That's about ten minutes from now." Grinding his teeth my friend scowled towards the mercenary. "Hey you!" The mercenary looked up. "Yes you! We could shoot you like a rabbit, you know. But we don't because you are different from your fascist friends."

The mercenary glared back at Hama with black hatred in his eyes.

"Hama, no good will come of this sort of talk," Serwan hissed in his ear.

"I just pray he never takes up arms against his own people again."

Everyone looked towards me. Had I just said that out loud? Apparently so. The mercenary locked his gaze with me.

"Brother doctor," he said solemnly. "By God, I will never do that again – never!"

Our expressions softened in unison, transforming from those of bitter rivals into those of resigned and resolute brethren.

"You should go home now, kaka," I told him quietly.

The man left without another word. He never looked back; he just headed behind the nearby hills and disappeared forever.

Now it was decision time for the rest of us. For me there was no decision to make. There was no way I was turning myself over to the Baghdad regime. And I hadn't entirely given up hope that the Pesh Merga would continue to fight on. I kept thinking that Iraqi Kurdistan was a vast labyrinth of wild mountains and invisible valleys where extensive forces could remain concealed indefinitely. But at the same time I understood that if the legendary Barzani had conceded then the revolution no longer had any leadership. I had to head back to Pen Jewin and find Kurdo. When I knew what his plans were, what his thoughts were, then and only then could I make further decisions. But somehow this would mean taking the patients currently under my care with me. How could I find reliable transportation for at least fifty people? I knew there was a land-rover prepared to take me, but at the most it held only twenty.

"Serwan, how do I choose who to take?" I asked desperately.

He didn't get a chance to answer before the first huge explosion rocked the ground under our feet. It sounded like the collective scream of all the lost souls in Kurdistan. The mountains themselves seemed to be weeping as they scrutinized the poor little children beneath them, dwarfed in both stature and significance as a people lost in the mists.

A second explosion.

I thought back to my time in Western civilization. I remembered a news report of a maniacal madman who had shot his family and set fire to his home just because he thought he had financial problems. How little he understood of what problems really were.

"We will have to burn everything," I heard someone say.

I couldn't focus properly through the stinging tears that washed clean tracks of salty water down my flushed and muddy face. Who had said that?

"Hama?"

"Yes, kaka doctor. We will have to burn everything – even ..."

"Even the hospital," Serwan finished his thought.

I felt sick. I felt physically, emotionally, and spiritually sick.

"But all the injured and crippled patients," I complained.

"We're retreating, brother doctor," Hama reminded me. "We can't leave anything behind for the enemy – not even your hospital."

A slow motion montage played through my mind of the time we'd had to dig out two tons of dung and fumigate the old stable, of the huge rocks we'd had to chip away a piece at a time to hide our new facility in the hillside, of the poor mules who had carried steel doors from a deserted city to keep out the grueling snows of winter. And now I had to destroy it? How could this be? What sort of madness was this? It was the final insult, the salt harshly thrown into the open and festering wound that was my heart – a heart shattered into so many pieces that no medical doctor could ever fix it.

"I can't do it," I wept. "I can't make the decision to destroy the hospital."

"Then someone else shall have to do it for you, brother doctor," Serwan said softly.

A short letter was written to the local Party headquarters. Ninety minutes later a reply was in my hands. In brief I was ordered to distribute what I could among the villagers and burn the rest. Everything had to be destroyed: the generator, the medical supplies, even my gynecological table. It all had to be gone, and so did we. We had until midnight.

My patients. How did I break the news to my patients? There was only one way: quickly. Like ripping a sticky plaster off sensitive flesh, the faster it was done the less you hoped it would hurt. I washed my face, cleared my throat and straightened my back. Taking a deep breath I walked into my cherished facility and tried to speak. At first the words wouldn't come up. "Get a grip," I told myself firmly. It had to be done...

"I have to inform you the revolution has broken down," I said authoritatively. "Barzani has asked the people to follow him into Iran."

"By God, I can't believe it," one of the Pesh Merga cried.

"It is true, kaka. The Shah has sold us out, and Barzani has accepted the decision."

"Just like that?"

"Just like that."

"It isn't true," Darwish shouted. "The situation is more complicated than that."

"We don't have time to explain," I hissed. "The mercenaries might take the area by nightfall."

"You mean all the brigades, all the Pesh Merga have decided to drop their weapons?" the Pesh Merga asked.

"We were given no time to think about it," Hama explained. "Until yesterday the leadership claimed the fight would continue, they said we could depend upon ourselves. But then the telegram came. The leadership never really intended to resume fighting after the truce expired. It had already conceded to the Shah's demands. It didn't announce its real intentions until the last moment to prevent a rebellion against their decision. If we'd had time we could have organized a new leadership. But now there is no time."

Hama had explained it very well. It was a fixed game from the start. What absolute betrayal! What useless loss of life! What tragedy!

"I would rather be hanged by the Ba'ath than live as a refugee in Iran," the Pesh Merga growled.

222

"No one is going to force you to go to Iran," I assured him.

"Kaka doctor," he said sadly. "Even if I did want to go to Iran, I can't make it on foot, I have no money for mules, and the car won't make it through the muddy mountains."

Another Pesh Merga continued his thought. "We should try and reach our own village, where our people can care for us until our injuries are healed."

"Is that what you want to do?" I asked them.

After glancing at each other fleeting, "Yes," they answered as one.

I nodded understandingly.

"We'll need some medicines and an official discharge letter."

"What the hell do you need an official discharge letter for?" Hama demanded.

"Kaka," the Pesh Merga shrugged. "You never know. Maybe it's all a trick, and if we leave our units without permission ..." he shrugged again, more expansively this time.

"If that is what you want, then that is what you shall have," I answered firmly. "I'll even give you all six week's leave."

"Brother doctor," Hama whispered to me. "If they get caught with a letter signed by you ..."

"To hell with it," I snapped back.

Making one final intensive tour of the wards, I put fresh bandages on the wounds, and told the orderly to make a list of medicines that each patient needed. Everyone was crying. Children cried because their mothers were crying. My staff were crying at all the blood, sweat and tears we'd shed for nothing. Even some of the Pesh Merga were crying. But I didn't cry. Not this time. Not yet. They would be plenty of tears to shed later.

When I returned to my living quarters I could see a huge crowd silhouetted against the fire-red hues of a blazing sunset. The intense blood reds and the blistering tinges of tangy orange dropping behind the lush green hills and the immense rugged mountains seemed to mimic the inferno that was yet to be lit. The people all stared at me in stunned silence as though they expected me to make some kind of announcement. I couldn't shake the thought of how these gallant people had been humiliated. A well-organized machinery of petty bourgeoisie in Algiers had sold them out for their own greed as easily as feuding landlords would transfer ownership of a flock of cattle.

"I have decided to head to Iran," I said suddenly.

Silence.

"From there I will try to leave the Middle East as quickly as possible. I will not surrender to the fascist Iraqi government, not even if I did believe they would show mercy. On both sides of the border there is evil. It is hard to decide which is the lesser. So my decision is to get to the outside world and tell the story, for only when those outside our borders learn the truth can we ever truly be free. But I make this promise to you now. I will come back. I will come back a free man, when all of Kurdistan is free!"

"By God, we are all with you, kaka doctor," one of the villagers cried out.

As I write this book Iraq is only now, in 2005, tasting the first sweet morsel of the freedom that I dreamed of over thirty years ago. Three long decades have passed since I made that speech, and all this time I have had to remain silent, for although I was free my family remained under the unrelenting subjugation of Ba'ath Party rule. Not one single second has ticked by during those thirty years without the memory and images of those parting moments haunting me. But throughout all that time a candle has burned in my heart for those people. It might have been a small candle, but its flame was eternal and in some meager way it helped me hold onto the belief that within its flickering light there was still hope. For me it was a glimmering wisp of a memory that would keep the proud people of Kurdistan alive and out of the dark.

That flame.

That candle.

The fire ...

It had to be done, but I couldn't watch. Perhaps that was cowardly of me, I don't know, but I couldn't be the one who lit the match. It was Ahmed who broke the news to me, blustering into my modest room tired, dirty, and sweaty.

"All that medicine," he gasped. "I can't believe it. How we fought to obtain it and now it's been thrown on a bonfire like garbage. The penicillin vials are exploding like hand grenades."

"And the hospital?" I stammered.

He paused.

"It has been dowsed in gasoline."

I sat in numb silence, wondering what would happen if the nearby trees caught fire. We could destroy hundreds of acres of vineyards, and with them the last shred of a means of survival for what remained of the village.

I don't know who it was that lit the flame. I didn't want to know. I still don't want to know. If ever I meet that person again I couldn't look them in the eye knowing, even though they had no choice, they were responsible for annihilating my humble yet vital hospital.

By seven o'clock that night the whole of Azad seemed to be ablaze. The smell of burning rubber from vehicle tires was almost asphyxiating. The crackle and pop of flames hungrily gorging themselves on the few measly possessions these people owned was nauseating to my sensibilities. The roasting heat from the surrounding infernos could surely have melted all the snow in Kurdistan; those malevolent, ravenous, ferocious flames that feasted without conscience or remorse as if sent directly from the very depths of hell. Yet all of this paled into insignificance for me when I thought of my noble little hospital blazing in radiant glory, when I thought of all the suffering patients I would no longer be able to care for, and when I though that if man could only learn to get along with fellow man none of this would ever have happened in the first place. I couldn't look. I couldn't cast my eyes upon such infernal calamity. Perhaps if I didn't look it wouldn't be true. Perhaps if I did look my eyes would be gouged out of their sockets for witnessing such wickedness. I couldn't look.

CHAPTER EIGHTEEN

"How are you going to get to Pen Jewin?" Ahmed asked me.

"The same way I came here – on foot."

"But kaka doctor, you'll never make it. It's not safe any more."

I allowed my eyes to soak in the image of my faithful friend with a heartrending weight that reached down into the depths of my soul.

"Kaka Ahmed, over one hundred people have decided to come with me. There is no other way for so many of us to travel but by foot."

My group was the last of those leaving the village. As though still attached to my beloved Azad by an invisible umbilical cord, I tried to savor each precious second I remained before I was severed from my people, perhaps forever. We ate no dinner that night. We drank black tea, and we smoked, but no one ate. The thought of one hundred souls traveling with me was overpowering. I didn't believe all these people should turn and leave their homes, so before I departed I decided there was one last thing I could attempt to avert this catastrophe. An old man by the name of Haji Ali was still in town. I needed to speak with him privately.

"Shall I tell him to come here?" Ahmed asked.

"No, my friend. I shall meet him outside by the stream."

Ahmed nodded. He seemed to understand I wanted to absorb what remained of the unspoiled natural beauty of our proud little village, like a dried-out thirsty sponge, before I said farewell. A short while later I found Haji, as I knew I would, standing by the stream, holding his rifle, and lighting a cigarette.

"Haji Ali," I said softly. "I know many of you are planning to head to Iran because that's what the leadership wants."

226

"We've been working for the hospital," he explained simply. "We have no choice. We all remember what happened in 1969. The mercenaries took over the conquered areas and shot every last man where they stood."

"But you will be leaving your families behind. How will they cope?"

"At least they will have a roof over their heads," he rasped in a trembling, broken voice. "I don't think the government will harm helpless women and children."

"But all you have done is help victims from both sides. You have done nothing wrong."

"You seem to forget that both the Ba'ath regime and the mercenaries are incapable of distinguishing between right and wrong. To them we have worked for the revolution. That is quite sufficient for them to hang every last one of us."

The reality of those words hung in the air as I lit two fresh cigarettes, one for each of us. I firmly believed it was no safer for these people to submit to Iranian regime than it would have been for them to surrender to the Ba'athists. And I knew if Haji Ali changed his mind, others would follow as he was considered a wise old sage of the village. But before I could formulate an intelligent reply, he surprised me.

"The rumor is that we'll resume the battle after a few months of regrouping. We'll come back even stronger."

"Those are just rumors. Barzani and his people are powerless now. With this treachery between Iran and Iraq he has no influence to help us. In two weeks the borders will be closed and everyone in Iran will be a refugee with no rights. And who knows what the Shah will do after that?"

"You mean he might send us back?"

"If he thinks it's in his interest."

"Then why are you going to Iran?"

"My situation is different. I'm a doctor. It's likely I would be able to leave quickly. Besides who could take the risk of hiding me here? Could you?"

"I tell you, kaka, either way we are lost."

That sounded to me as though he was beginning to change his mind. Perhaps I had said something intelligent after all. In my heart-of-hearts I honestly believed that the only chance these people had was to remain in passive defiance of all attempts to oust them.

"I can't make people change their minds," he added. "But I will talk to them."

"If we are to stand a chance in the future it will depend on the people who have remained behind. This is your land and these are your homes. You have the right to live here as free people. Tell me what last things I can do to help before I leave."

"We'll need food, but I don't want to take food from the revolution."

"What belongs to the revolution belongs to the people. I will get you the food you need."

"I will go and talk to my people," he said quietly, hurrying off.

Only then did a dark shape emerge from the shadows. One of my Pesh Merga friends had been listening to the conversation, intrigued to learn which way Haji Ali was going to swing.

"I agree handing ourselves over to the Shah might not be the most intelligent move," he said slowly. "Besides, I wouldn't go without my family, and I don't have enough money to pay for mules to carry seven children."

"So what are you planning to do?"

"I have decided to turn myself into the Susei garrison," he choked, starting to cry.

"Why?"

"It makes no difference any more. I am dead either way. Perhaps this way at least my family will stand a chance of survival."

"Kaka, there must be another way."

"No, kaka doctor. My mind is made up. This is what must be done. Goodbye my brother – and my friend."

We embraced firmly, neither one of us wanting to let go. The sound of our weeping mingled with the babbling of the gentle stream, resonant in a melancholy echo that was inaudible over the sound of the raging firestorm around us.

The night sky was rich with flames leaping in the ecstasy of their freedom – their freedom and our doom. Even the books that had found their way into the village were burning. And still I had neither the stomach nor the heart to cast my eyes upon the cremation of my hospital. I hadn't slept in three days, and I hadn't eaten in over twenty-four hours, yet I felt neither tired nor hungry. I was fired with the adrenalin of a man whose death-row sentence was about to be carried out. In the minutes before I finally left Azad my entire worldly possessions amounted to a briefcase that was so small it wouldn't even contain my three books of notes – so I burned those too. All I had left after that were the muddy khaki clothes I'd arrived in earlier that day. When the sun had risen that morning there was no doubt in my mind that we'd be moving the hospital and the battle would continue. What a difference a day makes! God Almighty, had it only been less than twenty-four hours? It felt like several lifetimes.

Hama stood looking at me, his bottom lip quivering. This was not farewell, it was goodbye. We embraced, we cried on each other's shoulders, and we parted, incapable of speaking a single word.

At least Haji Ali had done a good job. From over one hundred people traveling with me, we were down to a mere seven, including Serwan. It never ceased to amaze me how these people could play 'follow the leader'. At midnight we gathered around what was left of our headquarters feeling we might be the only people left alive in the whole world. The village had fallen deathly silent. Not even the dogs dared to bark; they didn't so much as whimper. We had truly become strangers in a strange land. The only sound was the roaring of the flames that maintained their ravenous rampage on all we had once called home.

Heading off in formation down the narrow road towards Yach-Samer, I couldn't contain myself any longer. As Lot's wife could not resist the temptation to look back when they left Sodom and Gomorrah, I had to look back. I had to see it. If I met with a fate similar to that in the legendary Biblical tale that saw Lot's wife (who had been warned not to look back) turned into pillar of salt for daring to defy her God, then so be it. I had to see my valiant little hospital one last time.

229

The full wrath of Satan himself was consuming my precious infirmary with an inferno so shamelessly full of vehemence I would swear the flames were trying to singe the gates of Heaven. The entire mountain behind it seemed to be ablaze. If I didn't know better I could have been convinced the shooting flares were on a direct trajectory to wound God.

I fell to my knees and wept like I had never wept before.

"Come, kaka doctor," a soft voice said to me kindly. "We have to go now."

∞∞

During our long journey to Pen Jewin we came across hundreds of people, some ready to surrender to the government, some heading for Iran, and even a Pesh Merga battalion leader who was rounding up as many people as he could to capitulate, thinking this might curry him some favor with the central command. Later I learned the more sickening reality of what the Ba'ath Party's idea of 'amnesty' was. One of three grisly fates awaited those who voluntarily surrendered: instant death, torture and imprisonment, or deportation to southern Iraq with their families where they were interned in concentration camps.

No one knew where the muddy roads were taking us as we left Azad on that fateful night, the falling rain mocking us with every step. I wondered how it could be raining when our souls were starved of salvation. Rain had always been seen as a symbol of abundance and goodness for the Kurds, but today the raindrops were bitter tears of acid. I saw mules pass us with three little children tied to their backs, looking like three little wet French poodles. Unwittingly I found myself wondering if they would ever grow up to have children of their own. There were a few brief moments of hope as we journeyed from my beloved Azad for the last time. En route we heard rumors that the remaining Pesh Merga had rallied their forces and were going to start the battle all over again, but as always with rumors, they were false.

230

I was amazed at the sheer volume of people who were prepared to surrender to the government, although the sentiment had probably been summed up best with the statement, "I'd rather be hanged here, than be a refugee there."

When we arrived in the village of Jach-Samer under a moonless sky there was deathly silence. Not a single light was on, not a single dog was barking. No candles flickered, no guards patrolled. Had we entered a ghost town, or were people asleep? How could anyone sleep on such a night? We headed towards an old mosque in the center of the village where a few bedraggled souls had gathered. We were tired and hungry and neither condition was about to be alleviated. We hadn't thought to bring bread with us, and the village had almost no food. I tried to get some sleep, but it was impossible. I just lay there, with my pistol under my head, seeing the image of my proud little hospital going up in smoke over and over again in my mind.

A few hours later I rose to a pale, dry morning and discovered my ranks had swelled to fifteen as a few Pesh Merga had decided to join us. We washed our faces and left hurriedly, without even thinking of breakfast. The sound of heavy artillery ricocheted in our ears from every direction, the sound of defeated Pesh Merga troops blowing up their ammunitions. Thirty years later the ricochet of those weapons still rings somewhere in the distant mists within my brain.

Crossing a rocky passage to wide green plains ahead I noticed a long column of maybe six hundred people walking in the opposite direction, led by a man astride a fine white stallion. My group immediately ran towards them, thinking they were armed Pesh Merga ready to restart the battle. When their leader spotted us he stopped his horse and waited. Breathlessly we reached this wondrous vision, hoping against hope that there was hope.

"Something new, kaka?" I asked urgently. "Where are you heading?"

"Nothing new," the leader said sadly. "It's just that we've all decided against going to Iran."

"What do you intend to do?"

"We are going home – going home to wait and see what happens. You can come with us if you wish. Our land is big, there is enough for everyone, and you would be welcome."

231

I looked at the man suspiciously.

"We have to stick together," he continued. "Near Mallomah there are more than ten thousand people gathered."

"Thank you," I said simply. "But we will continue to Iran."

"As you wish."

With those words he continued on his journey.

"Perhaps we should have gone with him to see what would happen," Ahmed suggested.

"I can tell you what would happen," I snapped disgustedly. "He's going to surrender to the government with his battalion, hoping it will save his skin." Quietly I clenched my fists in rage. "Come on. If we're to reach Pen Jewin before it's too late we don't have a moment to lose."

All around there were signs of the hopeless disintegration of a defeated and lost people heading towards a doomed fate. Our leadership had their backs to the wall. They were forced to capitulate with an unpopular decision, but over time the decision to capitulate was proven to be the correct one. Without a doubt it saved the Kurdish people from being utterly annihilated at that particular moment in history. In hindsight, had the war continued, the Kurdish people would have been fighting the combined forces of Iran and Iraq, an unthinkable situation that would have indisputably led to their complete and utter destruction down to the very last man, woman and child. In confusion, anger and panic at the time, people did feel that Barzani had betrayed them, however, history has proven his decision to be the correct one.

Wave after wave of people passed us silently with their heads down as though they were following their own funeral procession. Eventually it became too much for Ahmed. I turned to see him slumped under a tree crying.

"What will happen to us?" he wept. "I can't believe it's all over."

It was an impossible situation, an impossible choice. Ahmed was newly married and without his support his family was likely to be reduced to begging in the streets, if they survived at all. But if he went back he was dead. Either way he could not support his family.

"They will never forgive me," he sobbed, thinking of his young wife and daughter.

"I understand," I said sympathetically.

"Perhaps we should take the chance," one of my other traveling companions, suggested.

Without the benefit of a crystal ball to know which choice was better, or at least the lesser of two evils, I was not in a position to advise my friends. Both men ultimately decided to turn around. They took a side road through the mountains and sorrowfully walked out of my life forever. Another loss. Another piece of my soul chipped away into the abyss of epoch by the brutal futility of war.

Those of us who remained quickened our pace to the school where I had locked up food and medical supplies on my return journey from Pen Jewin the day before. Like slithering serpents we secured our hoard almost unnoticed, but it was for naught. Nowhere could we procure mules to carry the stash, not for love nor money. This presented more than one problem for me. Aside from needing transport to ferry the load, there was a river up ahead I would need to cross. As I was unable to swim, without a mule this crossing would be impossible for me. However, the impossible had been achieved before today. Unable to consider more than one dilemma at a time, I wrote a short note for the leader of a nearby village, asking him to send people to collect the medicines and use them as he saw fit. Afterwards I could do little but continue onward, praying that providence would provide me with a means by which I could cross an otherwise impassable hurdle when the time came.

With courage and determination failing, my group dwindled to just four: Serwan, Hama, a dresser from Baghdad, and myself. Nearing the village of Gapelon we noticed the explosions of ammunition supplies getting louder. Over a hundred Pesh Merga had gathered in a small yard in this village. It was quite a sight. Although numb in body and spirit I knew I had to find their leader, a Pesh Merga I knew well. I came across him inside a small hut, weeping like a baby, a broken man. It was pitiful, yet understandable. Every weapon he'd ordered destroyed had been paid for with blood. Each and every Pesh Merga under his command was precious to him. In any military action he was always the first to arrive and the last to leave. To witness his spirit broken was a travesty beyond words. When he told me his group had all decided to surrender, I couldn't believe my ears.

233

"Why?" I asked hopelessly. "Isn't there something we can do?"

I couldn't help wondering what would make a man volunteer for a death sentence. Was it shame and disgrace in the face of defeat? Was it indifference to everything, including one's own life? Or was it the vain hope that they might survive and be battle-ready when a mythical new struggle began?

"There is nothing you can do, kaka doctor," he said sadly. "We must surrender and hope the government takes mercy on our families."

I didn't have the mettle to ask him for assistance, it seemed as though I'd be offering a drowning man a glass of water. Overcome with grief I trudged outside.

"What did he say?" Serwan asked.

"Not much. He's going to surrender with his unit."

"Didn't you ask for some of the Pesh Merga to join us?"

"I couldn't find the words."

Just at that moment Hama came rushing towards us. "Brother doctor! I have just heard that the whole 1st and 5th battalions are near Kareza waiting for their commanders to arrive from Pen Jewin."

"Well," I breathed with the fresh air of new hope. "What are we waiting for? Let's go."

We turned to leave but hadn't taken three steps when a new surprise had our hearts standing still. All the Pesh Merga in Gapelon suddenly started firing their Kalashnikovs in the air, hundreds of deafening rounds at once. Customarily this was a signal of good news. Serwan dropped his bag and ran towards the Pesh Merga to find out what all the fuss was about. Hama and I blinked at each other in silent awestruck anticipation. Moments later Serwan raced back smiling broadly.

"You won't believe it," he gasped.

"What?"

"They say the fight will continue. The commanders at Kareza have brought the news back from Pen Jewin! Some of the Pesh Merga here are heading across the Kezlar mountains right now, to stop hundreds of people who are on their way to surrender."

"I don't believe it," Hama gushed.

234

"Believe it or not, it's true," Serwan insisted. "A unit is leaving right now to stop the surrender. The word has only just this moment come through on the radio."

"Impossible," I shouted.

Hama looked at me, amazed. "What did you say?"

"Nothing," I blushed.

"So, are we staying here or what?" Serwan wanted to know.

"I think we should continue to the 1st and 5th battalions near Kareza, and get the news straight from the horse's mouth."

"Sounds like a plan," Serwan cheered.

My little group all agreed. Kareza was only a forty-minute walk away, and mainly by a path of dry clay that presented relatively easy walking conditions for a change. En route we met a few other Pesh Merga who had all heard the same rumor. They added to our excitement by telling us they believed over a thousand Pesh Merga with commanders were gathered in Kareza. The news was heartening. Could it be true? Was there a chance after all? There was only one way to find out.

With a new spring in our step we seemed to reach Kareza in no time. Standing atop of a green hill my little band of determined collaborators looked down over a truly miraculous sight. There were indeed over a thousand Pesh Merga gathered in the beautiful tree-lined valley of babbling brooks below. It was a fantasy from a fairytale come true. Yet somewhere in the pit of my stomach was a nagging and disquieting sensation. It was an almost out-of-body experience, a sense of being on the outside looking in, despite being in the presence of so many noble partisans. A terrible feeling of loneliness engulfed me, as though a giant creature had swallowed me whole. None of my traveling companions noticed my black mood; they were too full of enthusiasm as this exciting sight. Yet as we scrambled down the hill to meet the commander of the 5th battalion I couldn't shake the ominous tremble of dread from my bones. When I looked into the commander's eyes his expression said it all.

There was no hope. His eyes were dead, hollow shells. I looked away, feeling somehow ashamed, and scurried around to find the commander of the first battalion. I knew the 1st battalion commander to be a younger man who may still carry a glimmer of hope.

235

Maneuvering my way through the mass of human misery I came upon the young Pesh Merga leader.

"What's the news?" I asked urgently.

"There's no news, kaka."

My heart sank.

"But they say the fighting's going to continue," I blustered, trying to sound optimistic.

"Just rumors. It's not true. I have just returned from Pen Jewin and I can tell you, kaka doctor, it's all over."

"Then why are so many Pesh Merga gathered here?"

"We have just dissolved the battalions, that's all. Now each man is free to make his own decision, but I'll tell you there is no way I am going to become a refugee under the Shah of Iran. I would rather be hanged here than die slowly there!"

I opened my mouth, but there were no words left inside me.

"What are you going to do, brother doctor?"

I shrugged, unable to meet his gaze.

"Brother doctor?"

"I'm going to Pen Jewin," I almost whispered.

"God be with you, kaka."

"And with you..." my voice trailed away as if a weight of immense proportions had just crushed what little was left of my soul.

CHAPTER NINETEEN

I think Serwan and Hama must have pushed me to continue after that overwhelmingly demoralizing encounter. I don't know; it's all a blur. I do remember a time later we arrived at a tiny village comprised of only a few houses. Incredibly the tea house was open, and even more incredibly the owner managed to find us some mules. Perhaps there was some good luck left in the world, perhaps the faintest glimmer of hope still did flicker somewhere on the distant horizon.

Among the spiritual and emotional pain we were all suffering, the physical agony of my shattered knee cartilage could almost have gone unnoticed – almost. Nonetheless, as painful as it was, I decided not to ride my mule until we reached the flooded river, giving the animal ample time to ready itself for the onerous burden of carrying me across the raging waters.

The sun sank lazily into a blazing horizon as we reached the dreaded river. I rebuked myself for the foolish fear of water I'd dragged along with me from childhood. I had seen more horror than I would have thought one mind could withstand, and for the most part I'd faced it with calm professionalism. Yet put me in front of a flooded stream and I'd fall to pieces. Then again, I reminded myself, the whole point about having an irrational fear is that it is just that – irrational! Anyway, I reasoned, it wasn't that irrational. I couldn't swim. If I fell off my mule I would drown, I would cease to be, I would die. I did not want to die! I wanted to live. I wanted to live and tell the world my story. And I wanted to live to see a free Iraq and a free Kurdistan. So actually my irrational fear was in fact entirely rational! Having wasted vital useless moments arguing with myself I discovered I was still unable to look this river in its face. How ridiculous! Look, for goodness sake, look!

A few furtive glances later the river seemed deceptively calm. Was that ease and calm I was beginning to feel? What truly strange times these were. After a final wrestling match with myself, knowing my options were to head forward over the river and face death by drowning, or head backwards to where the Iraqi army were proceeding rapidly on our position, suddenly the river wasn't quite as frightening. I would never surrender to the Butcher of Baghdad, never! I would rather face a thousand rivers than contemplate the torturous death and potential betrayal of my comrades which would certainly follow at the hands of my captors should I turn back. Besides, I decided if I were to fall off my mule I would just open my mouth so wide that the torrent could consume me effortlessly and swiftly, and I would have to worry no more.

Serwan and Hama swam across while I looked anywhere but at their aquatic prowess. Once they were safely on the other side with the mule owner I was instructed to remain calm. I scoffed to myself, "How does one remain calm when one isn't calm to start with?"

"Just remain calm," the mule owner called again. "Get on the mule, and let him do all the work."

Fine. I could do this. No problem.

Fully clothed, down to my shoes, I shut my eyes and climbed aboard the pony express to the other side of the river.

Oh, whoa! Did I say the river looked calm? I was wrong! As soon as my feet entered the water I could feel the surging current of raging waters surround me. If I fell off this mule no swimmer would be able to catch me at the speed I would be swept away. Roughly half way across the mule was pulled about forty meters to the left. Something innate in the animal seemed to be telling it there was no point struggling against this force of Mother Nature. I peeked out of one eye, then the other, and quickly realized if my noble steed didn't make his drive to the other side soon we would both be sunk – literally. I glanced towards my friends. Oh my God, where had they gone? I tried to call out, but the grating sandpaper in my throat prevented any vocal projection. It was clear what had happened. My friends hadn't moved. My mule and I had hit the marine equivalent of a jetstream that had surged us a great distance in the wrong direction.

Calm. Remain calm. No problem. More importantly, hold on tight! Don't let go.

"Argh!" I heard myself cry, as I was almost thrown from the creature's back. "Good horsey, come on, you can do it," I tried to offer encouragement. I'm quite sure some equine expletives were snorted in reply.

"Brother doctor, are you okay?"

Was that Serwan's voice? Cautiously I turned my head. I couldn't believe it. This gracious and courageous beast of burden had done it! Somehow he'd crossed the river and landed only a few feet away from my faithful friends. I was quite certain it was nothing short of a miracle.

"Serwan," I called back, rolling off the mule.

He raced towards me and I tried to stand, only to discover my legs had completely given way beneath me. Without the need for words we decided to take a short rest before attempting to continue our journey. My knee had virtually collapsed. I honestly didn't believe I could make it to Pen Jewin. Even after surviving the river crossing I was close to giving up, prepared to just lay there and die. And then it started raining again. Could it be any worse? I was afraid to even ask.

Alternating between riding the mule, which meant getting whipped by the full force of the freezing downpour, and walking behind the animal in excruciating pain, somehow I managed to move mile after mile in the direction of Pen Jewin. Up ahead were dark mountains with white peaks that we still had to cross before reaching muddy plains on the other side. I had never taken this particular route before. We were only taking it this time because it was deemed the 'safest' passage, that is to say least likely to fall under attack from the mercenaries. On one of our brief breaks I strapped my knee with part of my turban. Immediately there was some relief, a sense of warmth and firmness. I still had difficulty keeping up with my friends, but step after gritty determined step I edged closer to those mountain peaks. The higher we climbed, the colder it became. Our soaked clothes literally froze to our bodies, as icicles of precipitation pierced our exposed faces like sharp needles.

It took a Herculean effort, but finally we reached Pen Jewin, or what was left of it. The bustling city I had left only days ago had become a virtual ghost town. Pieces of destroyed weapons lay strewn across the streets. All the shops were closed. Every car we came across had broken down. Any hopes I'd held onto that I might find Kurdo here were instantly dashed. There was nothing for it but to continue to the center of town where we might find some transportation to Iran. At a garage in the middle of Pen Jewin three small buses stood crammed with what was probably the last of the town's population awaiting departure. A loud voice shouted out the fare and the regulations for travel. Whatever he was saying, it didn't register. Everything was a blur of nightmarish fantasy.

"Hey kaka," a young voice suddenly snapped me back to reality.

I looked down to see a wretched little street urchin.

"Kaka, would you sell your pistol?"

The pitiable child gazed up at me with a streetwise wisdom far beyond his years.

"There are no weapons allowed into Iran," Serwan reminded me.

"I will pay you a pound for it," the child insisted.

"You don't need to pay me," I said sadly, removing my ammunition belt. "You can have it as a gift."

"Wow! Thanks, kaka!"

I thought back to the time I'd been given that pistol as a gift from my dear friend, Hama. I turned to look at him. Hama gazed back at me with tears welling in his eyes.

"It's time for me to go now, brother doctor."

"Time for us all to go," I agreed.

"No, brother doctor. It's time for me to go back to my family in Azad."

"But I thought you were crossing the border with us into Iran?"

"No..." he let the word trail. "I just wanted to accompany you to the border to make sure you arrived safely."

"But," I began to protest. I was never to finish that sentence. The bus was starting to move. If I didn't climb aboard I'd be stuck in Iraq and face certain death.

"Hama," I stammered.

His teary eyes blinked their understanding at me. There was nothing I could do but climb onto that fateful bus, choking back the lump in my throat. I felt the mutual love and respect we shared for

240

one another wash over me as through the bus window Serwan and I watched Hama disappear at the end of the street, and the child rush off with his new treasure, removing the bullets from their holders and throwing the belt away. I only hoped this loathsome bounty brought him some good fortune. Certainly the fact that it was no longer in my possession was good fortune.

At the Iranian checkpoint two army officers boarded our bus, barking at us in Kurdish, "Anyone carrying a weapon must hand it to us now. If we find you are smuggling weapons when we search your luggage you will be automatically sentenced to death!"

So much for freedom in Iran!

Their search revealed no secret weapons cache and we were duly waved through across the border into Iran. Half an hour later I was heading towards the one hotel in town when a familiar voice cried, "Kaka doctor!"

Could it be?

I swung around.

"Kurdo!"

I ran to embrace my old friend.

"Kurdo, Kurdo! I didn't think I would ever see you again."

"Nor I you, brother doctor."

From the corner of my eye I could see Serwan watching us. Could I trust what I thought I saw? It seemed impossible. Through misty eyes clouded with tears, I swear I saw Serwan doing something rare among our people in these times of doom and damnation – he smiled.

"I hope we have done the right thing," Kurdo wept.

Standing back to look him in the eye I gazed soulfully at my friend, grateful we were both alive. "Only the future will tell," I said solemnly, as together we walked towards a brand new day.

EPILOGUE

Thirty years after I began to document this odyssey the world is a very different place. Many of the important players in this story are no longer on mortal coil; while others have gone on to achieve greatness. Among these are Jalal Al-Talabani, and of course the legendary Kurdish leader, General Barzani.

Jalal Al-Talabani played an important role in Kurdish politics for forty years. Since the overthrow of Saddam Hussein's regime he has taken the reins of Iraq firmly in his hands as the country's new President. He is also a man I am deeply honored to call my personal friend.

Jalal Al-Talabani was president of the Patriotic Union of Kurdistan (PUK) since the organization's founding in 1977. Born in Kelkan in 1933, he actively participated in the Iraqi Kurdish opposition from the age of thirteen, eventually becoming a central committee member inside the Kurdistan Democratic Party (KDP). He worked as a journalist and after the 1958 revolution commanded an Iraqi army tank unit. When the Kurdish rebellion began in 1961, Talabani became an active participant. Following the 1975 Algiers accords that led to the fall of the rebellion, Talabani split with the KDP and founded the PUK. Since the 1991 Kurdish uprising following the Kuwait war, the PUK has (along with Barzani's Kurdistan Democratic Party of Iraq) controlled parts of northern Iraq, claiming some four thousand men under arms. In Jalal Al-Talabani's own words:

"I don't see any future for Iraq except as a democracy. Democracy is medicine for all diseases. Iraq will not remain united unless it is democratic, because the social structure of Iraq requires freedom of expression, equality, and participation by representatives of all Iraqi

242

groups. This means democracy. Only democracy can offer all these options."

As for General Mustafa Barzani, who led the armed resistance against the fascist Ba'ath Party with his sons, no words can adequately express the depth of admiration and respect the Kurdish nation feels for this man. After he was forced into exile in Iran, when the revolution collapsed in 1975, Mustafa emigrated to the United States where in died in March, 1979. Millions of Kurds mourned his passing. He will forever be remembered in the hearts of the Kurdish people for supporting their struggle throughout his life. His memory continues to inspire Kurdish ideology as these people maintain their struggle for peace, freedom and democracy. Mustafa's son, Masoud, is the living embodiment of that vision as the present leader of the Kurdish Democratic Party.

Iraq has not overcome problems associated with its new constitution, with no full agreement yet reached between Shiites, Sunnis and Kurds. The Shiites and the Kurds look favorably on federation; however the Sunnis, who ran the country for years, are opposed to it. Masoud Barzani regularly speaks out on this subject, only recently saying that he prays to see an independent Kurdistan before he dies.

As for me, after I was reunited with Kurdo in Iran we decided to make our way to Teheran. We'd heard the Movement had established a headquarters to deal with the refugees pouring across the border, and luckily for me my younger sister had married an Assyrian from Iran. I will never forget the look on her face when I knocked on her door. The last time we'd met I was a strapping, healthy youth. The person my sister opened her door to was a complete stranger; a straggly, forty-seven kilo, shattered wreck. Once I convinced her I really was her brother, she and her husband looked after me well for the following two months I spent in Teheran.

Rumors began circulating that the Shah was going to return all the Kurds to Hussein's Iraq. Apparently the idea that so many educated Kurds might populate the free world disturbed the leaders on both sides of the border. Accordingly the Kurdish Movement recommended all refugees get exit visas from foreign embassies as fast as they could. Kurdo applied to Germany, Holland and Austria. I applied to Holland, Switzerland and the USA, thinking Germany would never take me back after sending me into exile following the Munich bombing. Ironically, as Kurdo didn't speak German, he asked me to assist in translating his meeting in the German Embassy. The General Consul at the Embassy was so astonished at my perfect German he began asking *me* questions. When he learned I was a German medical graduate, and the circumstances under which I'd left Germany, his shame and embarrassment were obvious. It was duly suggested that I apply to re-enter Germany.

Within two weeks I received a phone call from the General Consul confirming the rumors we'd been hearing about all Kurdish refugees being returned to Iraq. For my own safety (as Amnesty International had told this man I would be killed if I returned to Iraq) it was suggested I wait for my German visa in some other foreign country. Seeing the wisdom in this advice, I quickly renewed my passport and with help from both my Iranian brother-in-law and the Kurdish Movement in Teheran I secured a one-way ticket to Zurich. There I waited for my entry visa into Germany for the following three weeks, running out of money fast, and only able to eat every second day. All I could do was maintain a vigil at the German Consulate in Zurich asking the same question day after agonizing day: "Have my papers come through yet?"

Fortunately for me, I was one of the first to leave Iran. Many others were not so fortunate. Despite personnel in the Swiss office of the German Embassy being highly doubtful that a foreign national would receive an entry visa and work permit for Germany from outside of Germany, eventually the General Consul's promises from Teheran were honored. From that moment the formalities were concluded in ten minutes flat! With optimistic foresight, my brother-in-law and the Movement had made sure I was in possession of a valid ticket from Zurich to Stuttgart before I left Teheran. Finally I had everything I needed. As soon as my official papers were firmly in my grasp I was on my way back to my adopted home of Germany.

Within a week I was offered a job in the Veronika Clinic in Stuttgart as a ward doctor. Perhaps this was Germany's way of apologizing to me for the injustice of their hasty and ill-considered decision a few years earlier.

For the following twelve months I spent all night, every single night, writing down this story. I remembered every single second of the experience as though each incident had happened only yesterday. Every night I hammered out more notes with two fingers on an old-fashioned typewriter until my hands were too weary and my eyes were too bleary to continue. Only when I completed the record, twelve months later, did I realize I dare not publish it. Too many people I cared for were still living under the brutal rule of the Butcher of Baghdad. Any association with me and my record of events would have meant certain torture and summary execution for those I loved. For thirty long years I held onto my notes until Iraq was finally free.

My friend Kurdo was accepted by both Holland and Austria, and we remain in close contact to the present day. However, as I alluded earlier, not everyone was so fortunate. Hundreds of thousands of Kurds followed Barzani into Iran. Many of these were ultimately forced back into their villages to live under the grace of Saddam Hussein. Almost all of those poor souls met gruesome fates. From September, 1988, the Anfal campaign was carried out culminating in the destruction of four thousand villages and the disappearance of 182,000 Kurdish civilians.

No less than seven million Iraqis fled their beloved homeland during the tyrannical rule of Saddam Hussein, brethren who have now scattered to the four corners of the globe. They were the lucky ones.

Over a decade after I left Iran, I was sitting in my home in Germany when news broke about a day that has come to live in infamy, 'Bloody Friday'. This was the day when the whole world learned about the Kurdish people, and the diabolic lengths Saddam Hussein was prepared to go to.

MARCH 17th, 1988 …

In the township of Halabja, one hundred and fifty miles northeast of Baghdad, and ten miles from the Iranian border, the sun rose enthusiastically on what should have been a bright and peaceful day. Before the sun set again, five thousand of the seventy-thousand men, women, and children of the area lay dead, and a further seven thousand were injured. This was not the only chemical attack by Saddam Hussein, but it was most definitely the worst.

Chemical weapons and cluster bombs comprised of mustard gas, nerve agents, and cyanide were dropped on the unsuspecting populous amidst the infamous al-Anfal campaign where Hussein brutally repressed yet another of the Kurdish revolts during the Iran-Iraq war. These bombs were dropped not once, but twenty times.

Every murder destroys a measure of human dignity.

Every genocide murders a piece of the world as a whole.

The people of Halabja were burned as newly-grown plants crushed beneath a poisonous wind. In every street corner and alley, women and children rolled over on one another. The sound of children's laughter in liberated homes became the groan of despair for those who were fortunate enough to live to see the devastation.

It meant nothing that the Iraqi regime had signed the protocol of Geneva which prohibited the deployment of chemical and biological weapons in 1931. Nor did it seem to matter that the regulations of the 1972 Convention of this protocol requested all countries cease production, completion, and conservation of all kinds of chemical and biological weapons and demolish any stock piles they had. The 1972 Convention was accepted by all United Nations member countries, including Iraq. Hussein flagrantly and unashamedly ignored it.

No wounds, no blood, no traces of explosions were to be found on the bodies of his victims. Livestock and pets littered the crude earthen streets of this remote and neglected Kurdish town, having fallen to the same fate as their owners without discrimination or remorse. The skin of the bodies was strangely discolored; their eyes open and staring where they had not disappeared into their sockets, a grayish slime oozed from their mouths, and their extremities were grotesquely twisted.

This time the world media took notice. Images flooded living rooms across the planet of Halabja standing silent and deserted except for a lone dazed old man, absent during the bombing, who returned home to search for his family.

This poem by an unknown author perhaps says it best:

On the borders
Where throats are
Choked with good-byes
And eagerness is
Suspended in the eyes
And people asked
When ... where are we? And why?

Here a child dies.
There a baby lies, and
Another face-down cries:
My wound is hurting
My breath is hurting
My stomach is hurting
Mother: Am I to die?
And my white pigeon ...
Are we going to die?

In tears she said:
There beyond the border posts
Only days, we won't die
For us, God will try.

Again the child cries:
Will my pigeon die?
Mother: I love her
She is my life
Because I love her
She does not deserve to die.

All broke in tears:
Dear, your pigeon died
When the planes pried.
And she broke in tears:

My white pigeon was gassed?
My Kurdish pigeon died?
Mother! My hair is falling
Why? Am I to die?
Some water please ...
W-a-t-e-r ....

Human Rights observers estimated that Hussein's holocaust was responsible for the deaths of up to one hundred thousand Kurds in 1988 alone. The Nobel Laureate and WWII holocaust survivor, Elie Wiesel, said, "We have a moral obligation to intervene where evil is in control. Today that place is Iraq."

It has been said that the Kurdish people make up the largest stateless nation on earth. They have been widely despised by their neighbors for centuries. While they are mainly Muslim there are in fact Jewish and Christian Kurds, and even a few followers of the Yezidi religion, which has its roots in Sufism and Zoroastrianism. A Kurdish safe-haven only began to emerge in northern Iraq after the United States helped drive Hussein out of Kuwait in 1991. At that time President George Bush Snr ignored an uprising that he himself had stoked, which saw Kurds and Shiites in Iraq slaughtered by the thousands. Thousands more fled to Turkey, immediately creating a humanitarian disaster of dramatic proportions. The Bush administration, faced with a televised catastrophe, declared northern Iraq a no-fly zone, and thus a safe haven, a tactic that allowed the refugees to return home. Yet in 2001 the United Nations Commission on Human Rights found reason to condemn the Iraqi regime once more.

In 2001 it was said that an estimated three-hundred thousand Iraqi citizens had vanished without a trace. The UN Commission stated, "Widespread, systematic torture and the maintaining of decrees prescribing cruel and inhuman punishment as penalty for offences is commonplace. Torture methods have included hanging, beating, rape, and burning alive." The 2001 United States Department of State Human Rights Report said the Iraqi government, "killed and tortured persons suspected of – or related to persons suspected of – economic crimes, military desertion and a variety of other activities. Security

248

forces routinely tortured, beat, raped, and otherwise abused detainees."

U.S. Secretary of State, Colin Powell, told the United Nations that sources have said Iraq experimented on human beings to perfect biological and chemical weapons. "A source said that sixteen hundred death row prisoners were transferred in 1995 to a special unit for such experiments."

Mass graves excavated in northern Iraq revealed nine trenches including the skeletons of unborn babies, as well as toddlers still clutching their toys. The victims were believed to be Kurds killed in 1987/88, their bodies bulldozed after being summarily shot. The body of one woman was found still grasping her baby. The infant had been shot in the head, and the woman in the face. The youngest fetus to be unearthed was only twenty fetal weeks old with tiny bones no bigger than matchsticks.

There were those in the world who opposed the latest Bush Administration's 'war against terror' when once again the full fury of the American military machine went to war with the Butcher of Baghdad. Aside from those in the Western World who had their own reasons for objecting, there were people within Iraq itself who protested against this war. Those outside Iraq who would oppose the overthrow of one of the world's most hated men used the internal objections of the Iraqi people as means to justify their own positions of pacifism. However, those outside of Iraq perhaps did not understand why people within the regime's walls were objecting. These people were not pro-Saddam (for the most part) and they were not anti-American or anti-George Bush. They were just sick of killing and trying to avert a conflict that they thought would only lead to further suffering for the Iraqi people.

From where I stand, and from where ninety-percent of the Iraqi population stood, it was clear that the people of Iraq had no chance of freeing themselves from the Butcher of Baghdad without the assistance of President George W. Bush. Whatever anyone might think of George W. Bush, the fact remains that if he hadn't stepped in, Iraq would have suffered a hundred thousand years of subjugation under the brutal hands of Hussein and his sons. Time and again we proved incapable of liberating ourselves, so to President George W.

Bush I say THANK YOU – thank you from the bottom of my heart for ridding our country and the world of one of the most monstrously depraved, loathsome, foul, abominable, vile villains who has ever ruled on earth.

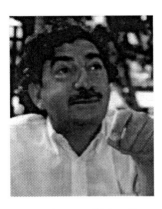

Dr. med. Albert Arkhim Gewargis

About Albert Arkhim Gewargis

Albert Arkhim Gewargis completed High School in Kirkuk, Iraq, passing the Baccalaureate State Examination before moving to Texas, USA, where he completed a Bachelor of Science majoring in chemistry. In 1963 he took up residence in Germany where he completed medical school at the University of Erlangen-Nuremberg. In 1971 he interned in surgery and urology at Kreiskrankenhaus Burgebrach, in the West German town of Bavaria. A year later he received his full medical license and worked as a surgical and ward doctor in Kreiskrankenhaus Pfarrkirchen, before leaving Germany late in 1972 to return to Iraq.

Working against Herculean hurdles in the Kurdish liberated north of the country, Albert remained in Iraq until the forced surrender of the revolutionists to the Ba'ath Party left him with no choice but to flee into Iran. When Amnesty International declared Albert would be killed if he returned to Iraq, the German Embassy in Teheran recognized the injustice that had been perpetrated on this remarkable man in his expulsion from Germany in 1972. By way of reparation the German government restored Albert's rights as a German resident by granting him an entry visa and work permit.

Returning to Germany in 1975 Albert again worked as a surgical and ward doctor, this time in the Veronika Klinik in Stuttgart,

251

Kreiskrankenhaus Kunzelsau, and Kreiskrankenhaus in Mutlangen. In 1980 he received his Degree of Doctor of Medicine (Dr. Med.) with a grade of 'Magna cum laude' and was recognized as a surgeon in Baden-Württemberg, West Germany. The following year he was licensed to practice as a doctor in his own surgery and registered a facility in Bavaria, where he continues to operate to this day. By 1986 this dedicated man of medicine was given permission to train young general practitioners in his private surgery, and in 1989 he was granted the recognition to bear the title 'General Practitioner' through the Medical Association of the State of Bavaria.

With the coming of the new millennia, Albert established the 'Doctor Gewargis Foundation' for special achievement by young students in the city of Luhe - Wildenau. In the latest of a string of honors and qualifications, in 2005 Albert was nominated and elected as an Honorary Citizen of the City of Luhe-Wildenau, Bavaria, per acclamation by the City Council – an honor that has for the first time been bestowed upon a foreign national.

Albert is a Member and Fellow of The Main Association for German Surgeons, the Main Association for German General Practitioners, the Bavarian Organization for General Practitioners, the Bavarian Association of Registered Doctors, the German Society for Ultrasound (DEGUM), and the Association of German Doctors (Hartmannbund).

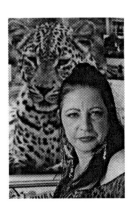

About Lynn Santer

Lynn Santer's first novel, *Sins of Life,* was the best-selling title for Minerva Press (UK) in 1999. Since then this prolific writer has written and ghostwritten thirteen books and twenty feature screenplays, including the controversial bestsellers *Land of the Free* and *Professor Midnight*. Hollywood veterans have optioned her feature screenplays and her short film and live theatre productions have won numerous awards.

Other books by Lynn Santer can be seen at:
http://www.lynnsanter.com

Printed in the United States
87389LV00002B/11/A

9 781921 118944